Vegan AIR FRYER COOKBOOK

200 DELICIOUS, WHOLESOME RECIPES

TO FRY, BAKE, GRILL, AND ROAST

FLAVORFUL PLANT-BASED MEALS

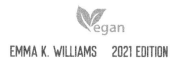

EMMA K. WILLIAMS   2021 EDITION

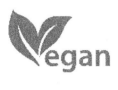

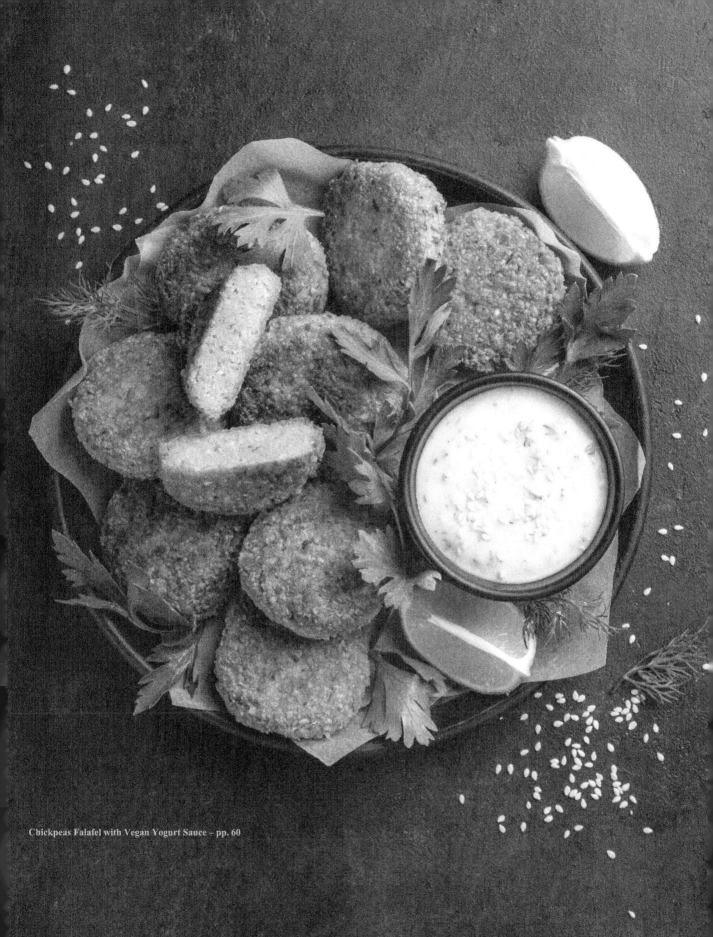

Chickpeas Falafel with Vegan Yogurt Sauce – pp. 60

CONTENTS

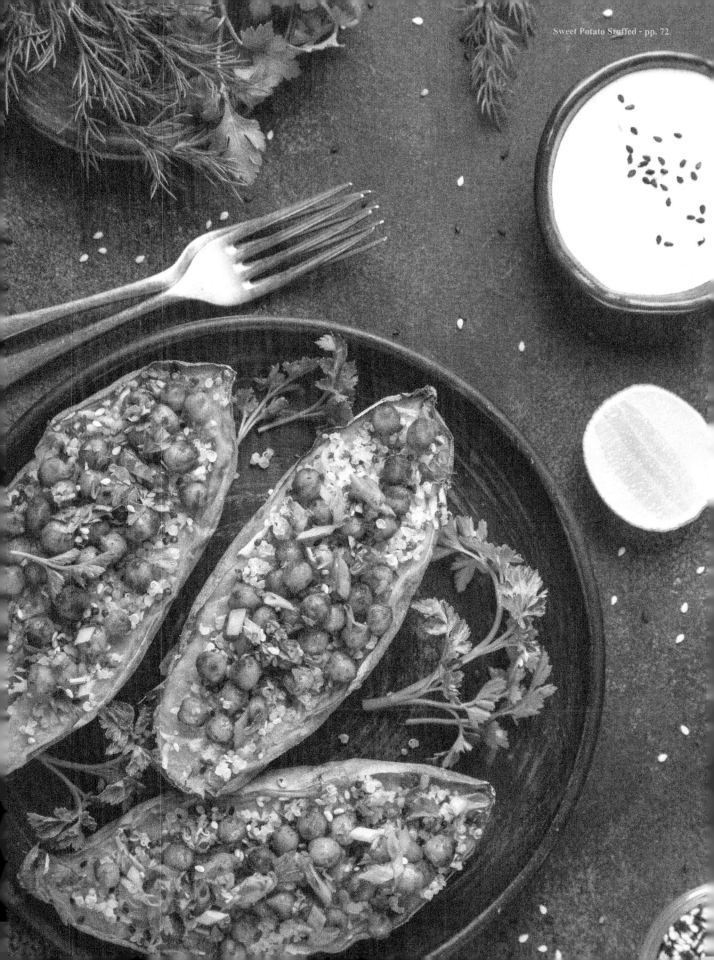

INTRODUCTION

Do you like the idea of deep-fried food? Want to be able to cook fries without oil? Yes, you read that right. You can now enjoy a multitude of fried foods without all the unhealthy grease, oils, and fats! Are you wondering how is this possible? The answer is quite simple - use an air fryer! An air fryer is similar to an oven as both appliances use hot air to cook food. But don't let the name fool you, you can do so much more than just frying. You can roast, bake, and even grill using the air fryer! You can make a variety of dishes such as ravioli and cookies in an air fryer. If you hate the idea of a cluttered countertop, this is the only appliance you will need to prepare flavorful and nutritious meals in less time. Forget about spending hours in the kitchen cooking and cleaning. Use, maintenance, and clean-up are simple and convenient. This book is a treasure trove of vegan recipes that can be made in an air fryer. You can now enjoy your favorite vegan dishes which you would otherwise deep fry to add flavor, without excess oil.

A vegan diet is 100% plant-based devoid of all animal products including eggs, dairy products, and honey. Going vegan might sound like a buzzword meant to make headlines, but this diet offers a variety of health benefits ranging from weight loss and maintenance, to better nutrition and reducing the risk of chronic health problems. Along with this, the vegan diet is environmentally conscious, sustainable, and ethical. An air fryer is a perfect appliance for the vegan diet and following a diet has never been this simple or delicious. This book is filled with vegan recipes suitable for using this fun groundbreaking appliance. Make sure you stock up your pantry with all the required ingredients. Just follow along with the simple and easy recipes I have found to whip up something delicious and nutritious restaurant-quality vegan food.

CHAPTER 1

AIR FRYER BASICS

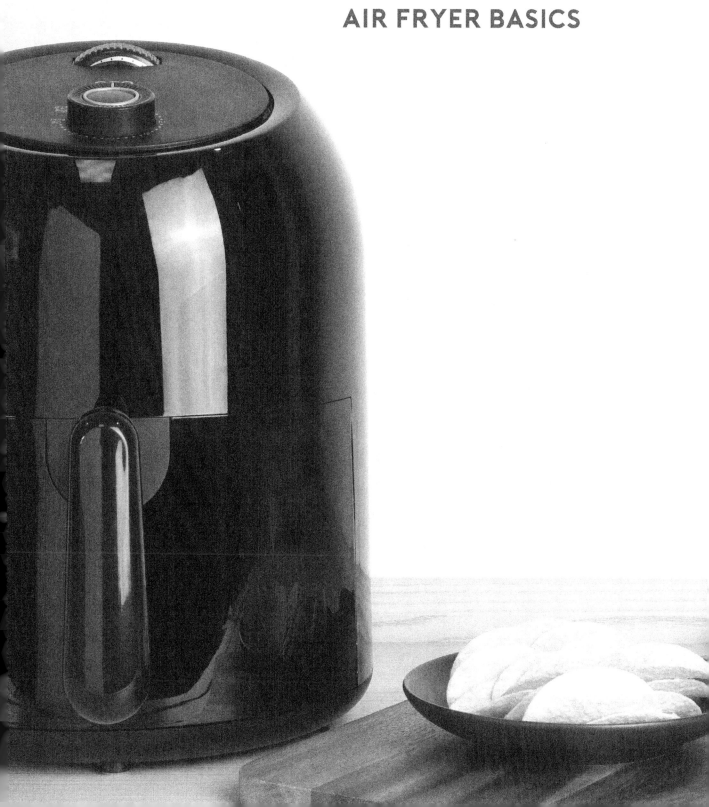

HOW DOES IT WORK

Air fryers have become a widely used kitchen appliance as they are a "guilt-free" and healthy way to enjoy fried food. This appliance has helped to reduce the fat content in popular foods, such as chicken wings, fish sticks, French fries, and even empanadas. Air fryers produce a crispy and crunchy exterior by circulating hot air around the ingredients. This circulation of hot air leads to the chemical reaction Maillard effect. This reaction occurs between reducing sugar and amino acid. It is through the effect that the flavor and color of the food change.

Since air-fried foods have significantly lower calories from fat, they are a much healthier alternative to fried foods. You no longer have to submerge your food in a pan filled with oil to get that taste you are looking for. To achieve a similar texture and flavor, you just have to spray a very small amount of oil on the ingredients before placing them in the basket.

Now that you know what an air fryer is, and how it works, let's look at the different ways in which you can use the appliance.

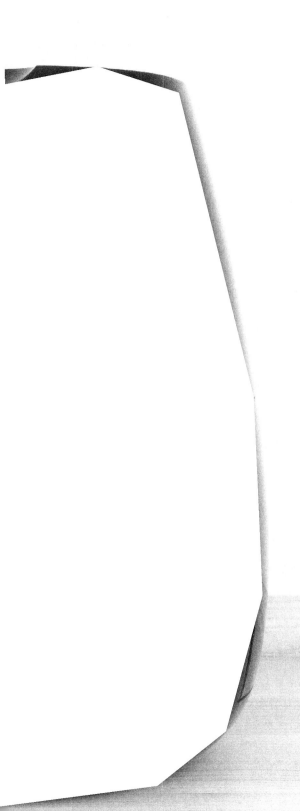

GRILLING

When you use traditional methods of grilling, you need to flip the item to get an even cook on both sides. You do not have to do this with an air fryer. You only need to prep the ingredients and place them on the grill layer or pan with a handle. The grill surface soaks up any excess fat in the food, which will leave you with a healthy dish. Shake the pan halfway through the cooking time to ensure the cook is even.

BAKING

Most people do not know that they can use their air fryer to bake. All air fryers come with a baking fan, which you can use to bake cupcakes, brownies, bread, muffins, and other desserts.

ROASTING

If you are too busy to make dinner, do not fret. Use your air fryer to roast meat and vegetables to prepare a delicious, nutritious meal. Using this appliance, you can roast to perfection faster than a traditional oven.

FRYING

As you might imagine, frying food with an air fryer leaves a crispy layer on the outside that gives you a good crunch while still being soft on the inside. An air fryer produces food that has 80% less fat when compared to the traditional ways. So you can still indulge in your favorite fried foods without feeling too much guilt.

BENEFITS OF AN AIR FRYER

REDUCES FAT CONTENT

Everybody knows that deep-fried food has higher fat content when compared to other types because of how they are prepared. For instance, a chicken breast roasted in an air fryer has 30% less fat when compared to deep-fried chicken. Some air fryer manufacturers claim that you can reduce the fat content in food by 75% when you use an air fryer since it uses less oil. Most deep-fried recipes require at least 3 cups of oil while air-fried foods only need one spoon of oil. This indicates that an air fryer uses 50 times less than the quantity of oil used in a deep fryer. The oil used in an air fryer is not absorbed by the food you place in the fryer basket, reducing the overall fat. Food cooked in an air fryer has moisture content and color like deep-fried foods (Teruel, M. del R., et al. 2015.). Further, the former is less fatty when compared to deep-fried foods. This impacts your health positively and reduces the risk of inflammation and heart diseases caused due to a high intake of fats.

PROMOTES WEIGHT LOSS

You already know that deep-fried foods are high in calories and fats that contribute to weight gain. A study conducted on Spanish subjects found that those who consumed large volumes of fried foods were at a greater risk for obesity when compared to subjects who only ate clean (Guallar-Castillón, P et al. 2007). Dietary fat contains at least twice the number of calories per gram when compared to other macronutrients, such as carbohydrates and protein. Since air-fried food is low in fat, it is best to switch to these foods if you want to lose weight or reduce caloric intake.

REDUCES THE FORMATION OF HARMFUL COMPOUNDS

Frying food in a lot of oil creates a lot of dangerous compounds, including acrylamide. This is formed when you deep-fry carb-rich foods. The International Agency for Research on Cancer stated that acrylamide is a carcinogenic compound. The agency researched to determine that acrylamide is linked to the growth and development of cancer cells. The results of this research are mixed. There is a significant association between acrylamide and an increased risk of ovarian, kidney, and endometrial cancers (Virk-Baker, et al (2015). When you air fry your food, you can reduce the number of acrylamides created by 95%. Some compounds, such as heterocyclic amines, polycyclic aromatic hydrocarbons, and aldehydes, which can be cancer forming, are present when food is cooked at high temperatures for too long.

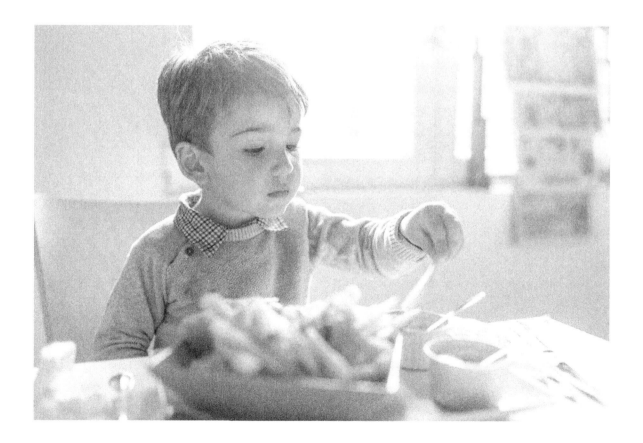

TOP 10 AIR FRYERS

MODEL	CAPACITY	FUNCTIONS
Ultrean Air Fryer	4.2 Quarts	• *Multifunction Cooker to fry, grill, roast, and bake* • *Easy to clean: dishwasher safe basket* • *auto switch off timer (0-30mins) and adjustable temperature setting*
Chefman TurboFry	2 Quarts	• *Healthy frying using at least 98% less oil than traditional fryers* • *Space-saving compact size* • *Easy to clean: dishwasher safe fryer basket*
Philips Premium TurboStar	2,75 Quarts	• *Fry. bake. grill. roast, reheat functions* • *Fat Removal Technology for healthy meals, fry with up to 90% less fat* • *Rapid Air technology with 7x faster air flow*
Ninja Air Fryer	4 Quarts	• *4 cooking functions* • *75 % less fat than traditional frying methods* • *Easy to clean: dishwasher safe parts*
Ninja Air Fryer Max XL	5.5 Quarts	• *7 different cooking settings, including air broil and max crisp* • *Air fry with up to 75 % less fat than traditional frying methods* • *Max Crisp technology*

MODEL	CAPACITY	FUNCTIONS
COSORI Air Fryer Max XL	5.8 Quarts	• *11 presets for popular dishes* • *85% less oil than traditional deep-frying methods* • *Digital display*
COMFEE' Digital Air Fryer	5.8 Quarts	• *8 preset functions* • *The hot air fryers oven can reduce 90% oil for healthy diets* • *User Friendly and safe to use*
GoWISE GW22956-7	7 Quarts	• *8 presets for popular dishes* • *Touchscreen display* • *3 dehydrating racks*
GoWISE USA 7-Quart Electric Air Fryer	7 Quarts	• *8 different cooking functions* • *Can cook large batches at once* • *Compact and sleek design*
Instant Pot Vortex Plus	10 Quarts	• *7 built-in smart programs, including bake, roast, toast, broil, dehydrate, and rotisserie* • *Deep-fried flavor with little to no oil for healthy meals* • *Easy to clean*

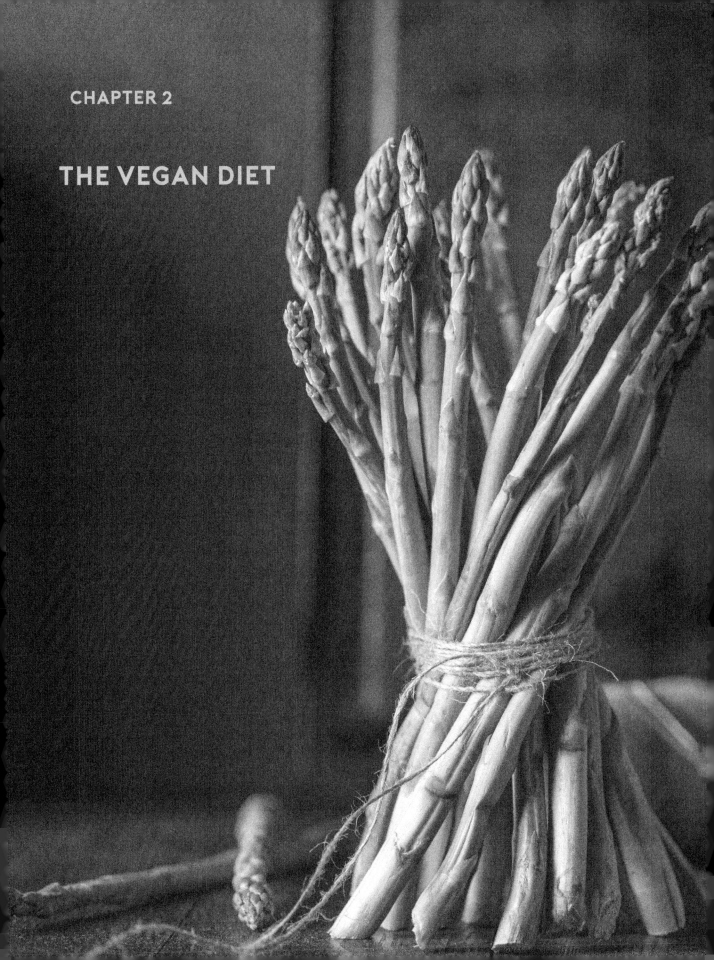

CHAPTER 2

THE VEGAN DIET

The most difficult aspect about being a vegan is not the transition from a meat-based diet but the fact that very few places actually cater to vegans. The best thing to do in such a case is to prepare your own food at home, especially healthy home-cooked versions of crispy snacks that are usually deep-fried. The air-fryer will make your life much easier in that regard. However, it is important to pay attention to your nutrient needs and not just focus on the taste and texture of your food. Whether you follow a vegan diet or not, it is important to eat whole grains, seeds, nuts, beans, and vegetables. Even if you include these foods in your diet, you may not meet the required nutrient intake. As a vegan, you must pay attention to the following nutrients:

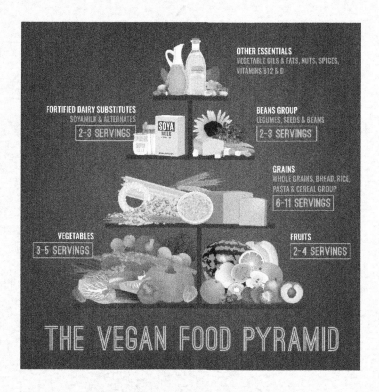

- **PROTEIN**
- **CALCIUM**
- **IRON**
- **ZINC**
- **VITAMIN A**
- **OMEGA-3 FATS**
- **VITAMIN B12**
- **VITAMIN**

Most of these nutrients are associated with various animal products and foods. As a vegan, you do not have to worry since most of the nutrients mentioned above, except for Vitamin D and B12, can be found in plant-based foods. Now let's give a deeper look at the list of nutrients you need as a vegan and which foods you should include getting overall nutrition.

PROTEIN

It is often said that as a vegan, you can maintain adequate protein levels in your diet if you consume whole plant foods and the necessary calories depending on your stature. Unfortunately, only some people show symptoms when their diet is lacking. If you don't consume the required quantity of protein, it can severely affect your muscle and bone health. Including high amounts of legumes in your diet increases the number of amino acids, such as lysine, which are the building blocks of protein. Nutritionists recommend that vegans should eat at least three servings of legumes every day. Include at least one of the following in each of your meals:

- *2 tablespoons of peanut butter*
- *½ cup cooked dried beans or lentils*
- *3 ounces veggie meat*
- *¼ cup peanuts or soy nut*
- *1 cup of soy milk. Alternatively, you can drink milk made from pea protein. Avoid other plant milk since they are low in protein.*
- *½ cup tofu or tempeh*

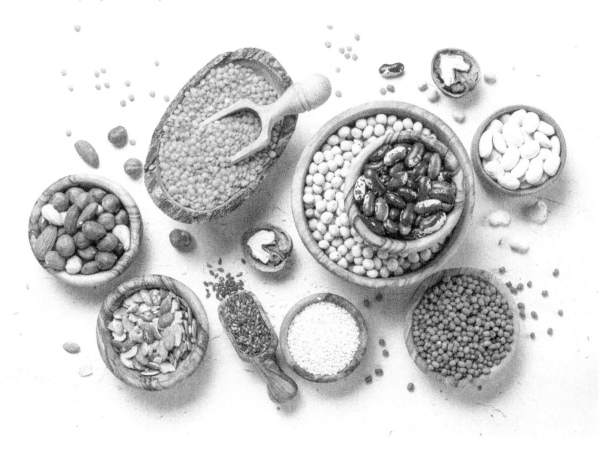

ZINC AND IRON

Beans and whole grains are rich in iron along with many other vegan options. Unfortunately, plant foods have compounds called phytates, which bind iron molecules to them making it hard for the body to absorb the iron from your food. Sprouting grains and toasting seeds and nuts make it easier for your body to absorb iron. Another way to improve your body's ability to absorb iron is by increasing your consumption of vitamin C. When you consume this vitamin along with iron-rich food, the vitamin breaks the bond between phytates and iron, which boosts absorption.

As a vegan, you need to eat enriched and whole grains, dried fruit, and leafy green vegetables. Increase your intake of vitamin C food to your meals, and some sources of this vitamin include citrus juices and fruit, mango, kiwi, cantaloupe, papaya, strawberries, pineapple, Brussels sprouts, tomato juice, cauliflower, cabbage, broccoli, and peppers.

Zinc is another important mineral you need to consume as a vegan. Some sources of this mineral include legumes, nuts, seeds, and whole grains. Zinc, like iron, is bound to phytates that reduce the body's ability to absorb this mineral. Vitamin C cannot help here, therefore, you need to find the right ways to prepare food, so your body can absorb this mineral. Sprouting legumes and grains increases your body's ability to absorb zinc.

OMEGA-3 FATS

Most vegans forget about a fatty acid known as alpha-linolenic acid (ALA) even with a healthy diet. This is an essential omega-3 fatty acid, which is only present in some foods. If you want to meet your daily requirement of this acid, you need to consume one of the following options:

- *1 ½ tsp chia seeds*
- *1 ½ tsp hemp seed oil*
- *1 tbsp of ground flaxseed (grind them to increase your body's ability to absorb the fatty acid)*
- *½ tbsp hemp seeds*
- *1 tbsp of walnut or canola oil*
- *1 ½ tsp flaxseed oil*
- *½ tbsp chopped walnuts*

The list is short, but these foods can help you meet your daily requirement of ALA. Add a few walnuts to your cereal or add a tablespoon of ground flaxseed to your meals or smoothies to make an impact on health.

CALCIUM

There was a lot of research conducted to determine the required quantity of nutrients every week and what you must consume. Experts believed that animal protein absorbs calcium from the body, which increased the requirement for people who consume milk, eggs, and meat. When further research was conducted, it became clear that protein protects bones, and your intake of protein does not impact your required calcium intake. It is important to consume the required quantity and pay attention to the type of food you eat since your body absorbs calcium differently from a variety of foods. For example, spinach is rich in calcium, but this mineral is bound to oxalates, which make it hard for your body to absorb the calcium. On the other hand, your body can absorb calcium easily from vegetables such as turnip greens, kale, broccoli, and bok choy.

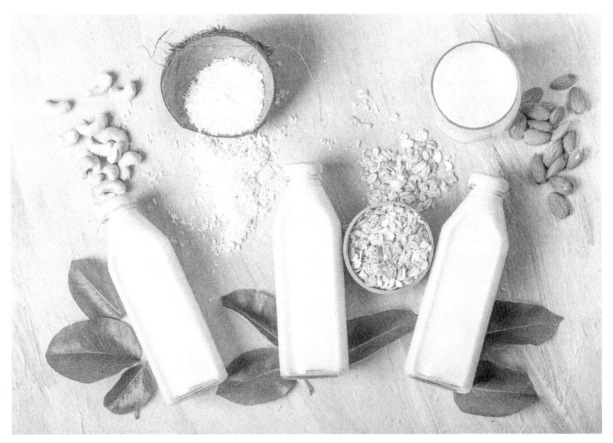

If you want to maintain your intake of calcium, you need to consume at least two cups of calcium-rich food each day. These foods include:

- *Cooked turnip greens, collards, mustard greens, bok choy, broccoli, and kale*
- *Calcium-fortified juices and plant milk*
- *Tofu with calcium sulfate8*

VITAMIN B

There is a lot of incorrect information out there on vitamin B12. Numerous websites claim vegans do not have to worry about their intake, but nutrition experts agree there are only two sources of vitamin B12 for vegans - supplements and vitamin B12 fortified foods. If you do not consume the required quantity of these foods or supplements, you can develop a deficiency. Fermented foods, organic vegetables, and sea vegetables do not have the required quantity of B12, so you can reduce the consumption of these foods. Nutritional yeast does contain a significant quantity of this vitamin, but only when it is grown on B12 media. If you are vegan or want to become vegan, you should absolutely consider taking B12 supplements. If you have a deficiency in this vitamin, it can lead to nerve damage and anemia. Always consults with a doctor before starting any supplement regimen

VITAMIN D

The body uses the sun to produce natural vitamin D. Clouds, sunscreen, and smog block the synthesis of this vitamin. When you expose your arms and face to the sunlight for at least 10 minutes a day, you can generate the required quantity of vitamin D. If you are unable to get the required exposure to the sun, you need to find a substitute. Vitamin D also is found in some types of fish and eggs, but the quantity present in these ingredients is quite low. This means most people, vegan or not, need to consume fortified foods or take vitamin D supplements to prevent deficiency. D3 is a common form of this vitamin found in supplements and various foods and derived from animal products. Vitamin D2 comes from the yeast, which is readily available in stores. If you have adequate levels of vitamin D present in your body, then the consumption of a supplement is enough to maintain healthy levels. Having said that, vitamin D3 is more effective to reverse a vitamin D deficiency. It is recommended that you consume at least 600 IUs of vitamin D each day.

VITAMIN A

Most vegan foods do not contain the required quantity of vitamin A, but vegetables and fruit have the required precursors to improve the body's ability to convert the nutrients into vitamin A molecules. These precursors include antioxidant beta-carotene, which is found in abundance in leafy and dark vegetables, such as spinach and kale. These precursors can also be found in carrots, sweet potatoes, and winter squash. When you consume one or two servings of these fruits or vegetables, you can take care of your vitamin A intake. You can increase your body's ability to absorb vitamin A from the foods you eat by drizzling a light spoon of oil, tahini, or avocado dressing.

7 TIPS TO MEET REQUIRED NUTRITION

CONSUME AT LEAST THREE SERVINGS OF TEMPEH, VEGGIE MEATS, SOYMILK, LEGUMES, PEANUT BUTTER, PEANUTS, AND TOFU EACH DAY.

INCLUDE A VARIETY OF VEGETABLES AND FRUIT IN YOUR DIET, ESPECIALLY DARK ORANGE AND LEAFY VEGETABLES. YOU ALSO NEED TO INCLUDE SOURCES OF VITAMIN C, SUCH AS CITRUS FRUIT, STRAWBERRIES, AND PEPPERS.

DO NOT CONSUME CONSISTENTLY OXALATE GREENS: SPINACH, BEET GREENS, AND SWISS CHARD. AN EXCESS OF OXALATE CAN RESULT IN A KIDNEY STONE.

INCREASE YOUR CONSUMPTION OF NUT BUTTER, NUTS, SEEDS, AVOCADOS, AND HEALTHY OILS TO MEET YOUR REQUIRED OMEGA 3 FAT INTAKE. CONSUME OCCASIONALLY, BUT ON A REGULAR BASE HEMP SEED, FLAXSEED, WALNUTS, OR CANOLA OIL.

CONSUME AT LEAST THREE CUPS OF CALCIUM-RICH FOOD EVERY DAY. INCLUDE FORTIFIED JUICES, FORTIFIED PLANT MILK, COOKED KALE, BOK CHOY, TURNIP GREENS, COLLARDS, AND TOFU MADE USING CALCIUM SULFATE.

DO NOT IGNORE SUPPLEMENTS, SINCE AS A VEGAN YOU NEED TO ENSURE YOU MEET YOUR DAILY REQUIREMENT OF VITAMIN B12 AND D. YOU CAN ACHIEVE THIS ONLY THROUGH SUPPLEMENTS.

LOW CHOLESTEROL CAN INHIBIT ESTROGEN OR TESTOSTERONE PRODUCTION. ALMONDS, PISTACHIOS, AND COCONUT OIL ARE HEALTHY FOODS THAT PROVIDE YOUR BODY THE RIGHT AMOUNT OF HDL CHOLESTEROL IF CONSUMED IN MODERATION.

MEN AND WOMEN

In this section, we will look at the daily intake of macronutrients for men and women. These numbers are relevant to men and women between the age group of 30 and 60 years, who weigh between 120 and 155 pounds.

MEN

- ENERGY – 2500KCAL
- FAT – 95G
- CARBOHYDRATES – 300G
- PROTEIN – 55G
- SATURATES – 30G
- SALT – 6G
- SUGAR – 120G

WOMEN

- ENERGY – 2000KCAL
- FAT – 70G
- CARBOHYDRATES – 260G
- PROTEIN – 50G
- SATURATES – 20G
- 1SALT – 6G
- SUGAR – 90G

Yes, the numbers are easy to follow, but how can you relate these to yourself? By personalizing your portions.

A   The portion size for carbohydrates, such as potato, cereal, rice, and pasta should be one fist. You can include one portion of these carbohydrates in your meal and ensure the food takes up only a quarter of your plate.

B   One portion of protein, such as pulses, beans, or tofu, should be the size of your palm. Try to include one portion in each of your meals.

C   The portion size for nuts and seeds is one fist, and it is best to consume these as a snack.

Now we will look at a wide range of vegan recipes you can prepare using an air fryer. There are more than 200 recipes, which will provide you ample variety to try out for every meal of the day.

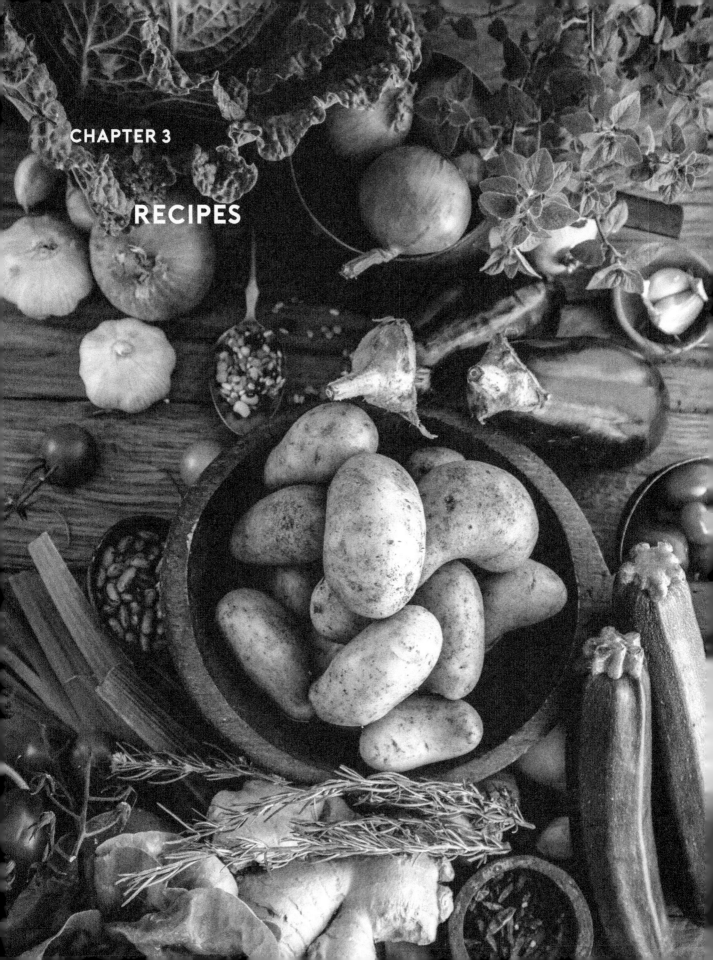

CHAPTER 3

RECIPES

BREAKFAST

*"Nothing will benefit human health and increase
the chances for survival of life on Earth as much as
the evolution to a vegetarian diet"*

— Albert Einstein

1. APPLE AND PEARS MIX

Ready in about: 25 min | **Servings:** 6

INGREDIENTS:

- 1½ cups coconut milk
- 1½ cups water
- 2 apples, cored, peeled, and chopped
- ½ tsp. cinnamon powder
- 1 cup steel cut oats
- ¼ tsp. nutmeg, ground
- ¼ tsp. ginger powder
- ¼ tsp. allspice, ground
- ¼ tsp. cardamom, ground
- 2 tsp. vanilla extract
- vegan cooking spray
- 1 tbsp. flaxseed, ground
- 2 tsp. stevia

DIRECTIONS:

Spray your air fryer with cooking spray, add apples, milk, water, cinnamon, oatmeal, allspice, nutme cardamom, ginger, vanilla, flax seeds, and stevia, mix, cover, and cook at 360°F for 15 minutes. Divide in bowls and serve.

2. BANANA AND WALNUT OATS

Ready in about: 20 min | **Servings:** 4

INGREDIENTS:

- 1 cup steel cut oats
- 1 banana, peeled and mashed
- 2 cups almond milk
- ¼ cup walnuts, chopped
- 2 cups water
- 2 tbsp. flaxseed flour
- ½ tsp. nutmeg, ground
- 1 tsp. vanilla extract
- 2 tsp. cinnamon powder

DIRECTIONS:

In your air fryer, mix the oats with mashed banana, almond milk, water, walnuts, flax flour, cinnamon, vani and nutmeg, mix, cover and cook at 360°F for 15 minutes. Divide into bowls and serve.

3. BLUEBERRIES OATS

Ready in about: 20 min | **Servings:** 4

INGREDIENTS:

- 1 cup steel cut oats
- 1 cup blueberries
- 1 cup coconut milk
- vegan cooking spray
- ½ tsp. vanilla extract
- 2 tbsp. agave nectar

DIRECTIONS:

Spray your air fryer with cooking spray, add oatmeal, milk, agave nectar, vanilla and blueberry, mix, cover a cook at 365°F for 10 minutes. Divide into bowls and serve.

4. CHIA PUDDING

Ready in about: 25 min | **Servings:** 2

INGREDIENTS:

- 2 cups coconut milk
- 1 cup chia seeds
- 2 tbsp. coconut, shredded and unsweetened
- ½ tsp. cinnamon powder
- ½ tsp. vanilla extract
- ¼ cup maple syrup
- 2 tsp. cocoa powder

DIRECTIONS:

In your air fryer, whisk together chia seeds, coconut milk, coconut, maple syrup, cinnamon, cocoa powder and vanilla, stir, cover and cook at 365°F for 15 minutes. Divide the chia pudding between bowls and serve.

5. CINNAMON OATMEAL

Ready in about: 25 min | **Servings:** 3

INGREDIENTS:

- 1 cup steel cut oats
- 1 tbsp. cinnamon powder
- 3 cups water
- 1 apple, cored and chopped

DIRECTIONS:

In your air fryer, mix the water with the oat, cinnamon and apple, mix, cover, and cook at 365°F for 15 minutes. Stir again, divide into bowls and serve.

6. CINNAMON TOAST

Ready in about: 15 min | **Servings:** 6

INGREDIENTS:

- 12 vegan bread slices
- 1 drizzle of vegetable oil
- ½ cup coconut sugar
- 1½ tsp. cinnamon powder
- 1½ tsp. vanilla extract
- 1 pinch of black pepper

DIRECTIONS:

In a bowl, combine the oil with the cinnamon, sugar, vanilla, and a pinch of pepper and mix well. This spread the slices of bread, place in the air fryer, cook at 400°F for 5 minutes, divide them between plates and serve.

7.   COCONUT RICE

Ready in about: 25 min | **Servings:** 4

INGREDIENTS:

- 2 cups almond milk
- 1 cup Arborio rice
- 1 cup coconut milk
- ¼ cup coconut flakes, toasted
- 2 tsp. vanilla extract
- ⅓ cup agave nectar

DIRECTIONS:

In your air fryer air, whisk together the rice milk, almond milk, coconut milk, the agave nectar, vanilla extract and coconut flakes, cover and cook at 360°F for 15 minutes. Divide into bowls and serve hot.

8.   CRANBERRY COCONUT QUINOA

Ready in about: 22 min | **Servings:** 4

INGREDIENTS:

- 3 cups coconut water
- 1 cup quinoa
- 1 tsp. vanilla extract
- ⅛ cup coconut flakes
- ⅛ cup almonds, chopped
- 3 tsp. stevia
- ¼ cup cranberries, dried

DIRECTIONS:

In your air fryer, mix the quinoa with coconut water, vanilla, stevia, coconut flakes, almonds, and blueberries mix, cover and cook at 365°F for 13 minutes. Divide into bowls and serve.

9.   DELICIOUS POTATOES

Ready in about: 45 min | **Servings:** 4

INGREDIENTS:

- 3 potatoes, cubed
- 2 tbsp. olive oil
- 1 yellow onion, chopped
- salt and black pepper to taste
- 1 red bell pepper, chopped
- 1 tsp. garlic powder
- 1 tsp. onion powder
- 1 tsp. sweet paprika

DIRECTIONS:

Grease the basket of your air fryer with olive oil, add the potatoes, sauté and season with salt and pepper. Add the onion, bell pepper, garlic powder, paprika, and onion powder, mix well, cover, and cook at 370°F for minutes. Divide the potato mixture between plates and serve for breakfast.

10. DELICIOUS PORRIDGE

eady in about: 26 min | **Servings:** 4

IGREDIENTS:

1¾ cups almond milk

3 cups brown rice, cooked

2 tbsp. coconut sugar

¼ tsp. vanilla extract

2 tbsp. raisins

2 tbsp. flaxseed meal

¼ tsp. cinnamon powder

RECTIONS:

, your air fryer, whisk together the rice, milk, sugar, flax flour, raisins, cinnamon, and vanilla, stir, cover and ok at 360°F for 16 minutes. Stir the porridge again, divide it into bowls and serve.

11. DELICIOUS TOFU AND ONION MIX

eady in about: 25 min | **Servings:** 2

GREDIENTS:

1 tsp. coconut aminos

vegan cooking spray

1 onion, sliced

¼ cup firm tofu, cubed

2 tbsp. flax meal mixed with 3 tbsp water

salt and black pepper to taste

RECTIONS:

ke a bowl, mix the flax meal with coconut aminos and black pepper and whisk well. Preheat at 360°F. Grease ur air fryer with cooking spray. Add onion slices and cook for 10 minutes. Add flax meal and tofu. Cook for ninutes more, divide between plates and serve!

12. EASY OATS

eady in about: 25 min | **Servings:** 4

GREDIENTS:

1 cup steel cut oats

2 cups almond milk

2 cups water

2 tbsp. cocoa powder

½ tsp. almond extract

⅓ cup cherries, dried

¼ cup stevia

For the sauce:

¼ tsp. almond extract

1½ cups cherries

2 tbsp. water

RECTIONS:

the pan of the air fryer, mix the almond milk with oats, water, the cherries dry , powdered cocoa, stevia and tsp. almond extract, mix, cover and cook at 360°F for 15 minutes. Meanwhile, in a saucepan, combine 2 p. of water with 1½ cups of cherries and ¼ tsp. of almond extract, stir, bring to a boil over medium heat l cook for 10 minutes. Divide the oatmeal between bowls, drizzle with the cherry sauce and serve.

13. PEAR OATMEAL

Ready in about: 25 min | **Servings:** 3

INGREDIENTS:

½ cup steel cut oats

2 cups coconut milk

½ tsp. vanilla extract

1 tbsp. stevia

½ tsp. maple extract

1 pear, chopped

DIRECTIONS:

In the pan of your air fryer, mix the coconut milk with the oats, vanilla, pear, maple extract, and stevia, m
cover and cook at 360°F for 15 minutes. Divide into bowls and serve.

14. PUMPKIN MUFFINS

Ready in about: 20 min | **Servings:** 2

INGREDIENTS:

½ cup pumpkin, peeled and cubed

1½ cups rolled oats

¼ cup maple syrup

¼ tsp. nutmeg, ground

⅓ cup cranberries

1 tsp. cinnamon powder

¼ tsp. ginger powder

DIRECTIONS:

In the blender, combine the oats with the pumpkin, maple syrup, cinnamon, ginger, and nutmeg and mix w
Add the cranberries to the mixture, pour the entire mixture into the muffin's cups, place them in the basket
the air fryer, cover and cook at 360°F for 10 minutes. Serve and enjoy.

15. PUMPKIN OATMEAL

Ready in about: 30 min | **Servings:** 4

INGREDIENTS:

½ cup pumpkin puree

1½ cups water

1 tsp. pumpkin pie spice

½ cup steel cut oats

3 tbsp. stevia

DIRECTIONS:

In your frying pan, mix the water with the oatmeal, pumpkin puree, spices, squash, and stevia, mix, cover a
simmer at 360°F for 20 minutes. Divide into bowls and serve for breakfast.

16. SIMPLE GRANOLA

Ready in about: 25 min | **Servings:** 3

INGREDIENTS:

½ cup bran flakes
½ cup granola

2 green apples, cored, peeled, and roughly chopped
⅛ cup maple syrup

¼ cup apple juice
2 tbsp. cashew butter
½ tsp. nutmeg, ground
1 tsp. cinnamon powder

DIRECTIONS:

In your air fryer, mix granola with bran flakes, apples, juice apple, maple syrup, cashew butter, cinnamon, and nutmeg, stir, cover and cook for 365°F for 15 minutes. Divide into bowls and serve.

17. SMOKED AIR FRIED TOFU

Ready in about: 22 min | **Servings:** 2

INGREDIENTS:

salt and black pepper to taste

1 tofu block, pressed and cubed
1 tbsp. smoked paprika

vegan cooking spray
¼ cup cornstarch

DIRECTIONS:

Grease the basket of your air fryer with cooking spray and heat the fryer to 370°F. In a bowl, combine the tofu with salt, pepper, smoked paprika, and cornstarch and mix well. Add the tofu to your air fryer basket and cook for 12 minutes, shaking the fryer every 4 minutes. Divide into bowls and serve for breakfast.

18. STRAWBERRY QUINOA

Ready in about: 20 min | **Servings:** 1

INGREDIENTS:

1 cup strawberries, halved
¾ cup water

¼ cup cashews
1 cup quinoa

1 stevia packet

DIRECTIONS:

In your air fryer's pan, mix the water with the cashews, quinoa, and stevia, mix, cover, and cook at 400°F for minutes. Add the strawberries, mix, divide into bowls and serve.

19. SWEET QUINOA MIX

Ready in about: 27 min | **Servings:** 6

INGREDIENTS:

- 1½ cups steel cut oats
- ½ cup quinoa
- 4 tbsp. stevia
- 2 tbsp. maple syrup
- 4½ cups almond milk
- 1½ tsp. vanilla extract
- vegan cooking spray
- strawberries, halved for serving

DIRECTIONS:

Spray your air fryer with cooking spray, add the oatmeal, quinoa, stevia, almond milk, maple syrup, and vanilla extract, mix, cover and cook at 365°F for 14 minutes. Divide into bowls, garnish with strawberries and serve

20. TOFU BREAKFAST

Ready in about: 24 min | **Servings:** 2

INGREDIENTS:

- 1 tbsp. oil
- salt and pepper to taste
- 1 tbsp. coriander seeds
- 1 tbsp. paprika
- 2 cups tofu
- 1 bay leaf
- 1 onion, sliced
- ½ cup lettuce, shredded

DIRECTIONS:

Grease a pan with oil. Add the tofu, salt and pepper, coriander seeds, paprika, bay leaf, and onion to a bowl Mix well. Pour into the pan. Bake in the air fryer for 20 min at 300°F. When done, top with lettuce and serve

21. TOFU SCRAMBLE

Ready in about: 35 min | **Servings:** 4

INGREDIENTS:

- 1 tofu block, cubed
- 2 tbsp. soy sauce
- 1 tsp. turmeric, ground
- 4 cups broccoli florets
- 2 tbsp. extra virgin olive oil
- salt and black pepper
- 2½ cup red potatoes, cubed
- 1 tsp. garlic and onion powder
- ½ cup yellow onion, chopped

DIRECTIONS:

Combine the tofu with 1 tbsp. of oil, salt, pepper, soy sauce, garlic and onion powder, turmeric, and onion in bowl, mix and set aside. In another bowl, toss the potatoes with the remaining oil, a pinch of salt and pepper and toss to coat. Place the potatoes in the fryer at 350°F and bake for 15 minutes, shaking once. Add the tofu and its marinade to the fryer and bake for 15 minutes. Add the broccoli to the air fryer and cook for another minutes. Serve immediately.

22. VANILLA PEAR OATMEAL

eady in about: 22 min | **Servings:** 3

INGREDIENTS:

½ cup steel cut oats

1 large pear, chopped

½ tsp. vanilla extract

1 tbsp. stevia

½ tsp. maple extract

2 cups coconut milk

DIRECTIONS:

Mix coconut milk, oats, vanilla, pear, maple extract, and stevia in your air fryer's pan. Stir, cover and cook at 0°F for 15 minutes. Divide into bowls and serve.

23. VEGAN CHEESE SANDWICH

eady in about: 18 min | **Servings:** 1

INGREDIENTS:

2 slices cashew cheese

2 slices of vegan bread

2 tsp. cashew butter

DIRECTIONS:

Spread the cashew butter on the slices of bread, add the vegan cheese in one slice, on the other, cut in half diagonally, place in the air fryer, cover and cook at 370°F for 8 minutes, turning the medium sandwiches. Serve immediately.

24. VEGGIE BURRITOS

eady in about: 20 min | **Servings:** 4

INGREDIENTS:

2 tbsp. tamari

2 tbsp. cashew butter

2 tbsp. water

4 rice papers

2 tbsp. of liquid smoke

½ cup sweet potatoes, steamed and cubed

a handful kale, chopped

7 asparagus stalks

½ small broccoli head, florets separated and steamed

8 roasted red peppers, chopped

DIRECTIONS:

In a portable bowl, combine the cashew butter with the water, tamari, and liquid smoke and mix well. Moisten rice sheets and place them on a work surface. Spread the sweet potatoes, broccoli, asparagus, red peppers, and kale, wrap the burritos and dip them in the cashew mixture. Place the burritos in your air fryer and bake 350°F for 10 minutes. Divide the vegetarian burritos between serving plates.

25. WHEAT AND SEED BREAD

Ready in about: 1 h 30 min | **Servings:** 4

INGREDIENTS:

1 tsp. of yeast

3½ ounces of flour

1 tsp. of salt

¼ cup of pumpkin seeds

3½ ounces of wheat flour

DIRECTIONS:

Combine wheat flour, yeast, salt, seeds, and the plain flour in a large bowl. Stir in ¾ cup of lukewarm wat and continue stirring until the dough is tender. Knead another 5 minutes until the dough becomes elastic a smooth. Shape a ball and cover it with a plastic bag. Leave to rest for 30 minutes. Heat your air fryer to air 390°F. Transfer the dough into a pizza pan and place it in the fryer air. Bake 18 minutes until it turns gold brown. Remove and place on a wire rack to cool.

26. ZUCCHINI OATMEAL

Ready in about: 25 min | **Servings:** 4

INGREDIENTS:

1 carrot, grated

½ cup steel cut oats

1½ cups almond milk

¼ tsp. nutmeg, ground

¼ zucchini, grated

¼ tsp. cloves, ground

2 tbsp. maple syrup

1 tsp. vanilla extract

½ tsp. cinnamon powder

¼ cup pecans, chopped

DIRECTIONS:

In your air fryer, mix the oats with the carrots, zucchini, almond milk, cloves, nutmeg, cinnamon, maple syr nuts and vanilla extract, mix, cover and bake at 365°F for 15 minutes. Divide into bowls and serve.

MAIN DISHES

*"Animals don't have a voice, but I do. A loud one. A big f*****g mouth.*
My voice is for them. And I'll never shut up while they suffer."

— Ricky Gervais

27. BEANS BURRITO

Ready in about: 20 min | **Servings:** 2

INGREDIENTS:

vegan cooking spray
2 cups baked black beans
½ red bell pepper, sliced
2 tbsp. vegan salsa

1 small avocado, peeled, pitted, and sliced
salt and black pepper to taste

⅛ cup cashew cheese, grated
vegan tortillas for serving

DIRECTIONS:

Lubricate your air fryer with cooking spray, add the beans, bell pepper, salsa, salt, and pepper, cover and coo at 400°F for 6 minutes. Arrange the tortillas on a work surface, distribute the bean mixture over each, also ac the avocado and cashews, roll the burritos, place them in the air fryer, cover and cook at 300°F for another minutes. Divide the burritos between plates and serve.

28. BELL PEPPER OATMEAL

Ready in about: 25 min | **Servings:** 2

INGREDIENTS:

2 tbsp. canned kidney beans, drained
1 cup steel cut oats

2 red bell peppers, chopped
¼ tsp. cumin, ground
1 pinch of sweet paprika

4 tbsp. coconut cream
salt and black pepper to taste

DIRECTIONS:

Heat your air fryer to 360°F, add the oatmeal, beans, peppers, coconut cream, paprika, salt, pepper, and cum mix, cover and cook for 16 minutes. Divide into bowls and serve.

29. BLACK BEANS MIX SOUP

Ready in about: 16 min | **Servings:** 2

INGREDIENTS:

4 cups black beans
2 zucchinis, chopped
3 onions, chopped

2 tbsp. olive oil
salt to taste
1 tbsp. oregano

1 tbsp. chili powder
½ cup green chilies
cilantro leaves to garnish

DIRECTIONS:

Add oil into the air fryer pot. Toss black beans, zucchini, onions, salt, oregano, chili powder, green chilies w salt. Cook at 300°F for 20 minutes. When finished, garnish and serve.

30. BLACK BEANS WITH LENTILS AND VEGGIES

Ready in about: 16 min | **Servings:** 4

INGREDIENTS:

1 tbsp. olive oil
1 red onion, chopped
2 carrots, chopped
1 tbsp. oregano

2 tbsp. garlic powder
2 tomatoes, chopped
1 cup water
1 cup lentils

4 cups black beans
salt to taste

DIRECTIONS:

Add oil into the air fryer pot. Combine the red onion, carrots, oregano, garlic powder, tomatoes, water, lentils, black beans, and salt. Cook at 300°F for 20 minutes. Serve.

31. BLACK EYED PEAS

Ready in about: 14 min | **Servings:** 2

INGREDIENTS:

2 sweet potatoes, sliced
1 tbsp. coriander seeds
1 tbsp. cumin seeds

4 cups black eyed peas
salt to taste
2 garlic cloves

2 cups tomato paste
1 onion, chopped

DIRECTIONS:

Add tomato paste into the air fryer pot. Mix the onion, garlic, salt, black peas, cumin seeds, and coriander seeds. Add the sweet potatoes. Cook at 300°F for 10 minutes. When it's ready, serve.

32. BROCCOLI AND MUSHROOMS MIX

Ready in about: 38 min | **Servings:** 2

INGREDIENTS:

1 broccoli head
10 ounces mushrooms, halved
1 garlic clove, minced

1 yellow onion, chopped
1 tbsp. balsamic vinegar
1 tbsp. olive oil
1 pinch of red pepper flakes

1 tsp. basil, dried
salt and black pepper
1 avocado, peeled, pitted, and roughly cubed

DIRECTIONS:

In a portable bowl, combine the mushrooms with the broccoli, onion, garlic and avocado. In another bowl, combine the vinegar, oil, salt, pepper and basil and mix well. Pour over the vegetables, toss to coat, set aside for 30 minutes, transfer to the air fryer basket and cook at 350°F for 8 minutes, divide between plates and serve with chili flakes.

33. BROCCOLI AND TOFU BOWLS

Ready in about: 25 min | **Servings:** 4

INGREDIENTS:

- 1 tsp. rice vinegar
- 1 block firm tofu, pressed and cubed
- 2 tbsp. coconut aminos
- 2 tbsp. vegan avocado pesto
- 1 cup quinoa, cooked
- 1 tbsp. olive oil
- 4 cups broccoli florets

DIRECTIONS:

In a portable bowl, mix the diced tofu with vinegar, coconut aminos, oil, and broccoli, mix and allow to stand for 10 minutes. Transfer the tofu to your air fryer basket and cook at 400°F for 10 minutes. Add the broccoli, cover the air fryer again and cook for another 5 minutes. Divide the quinoa between bowls, add the tofu and broccoli, top with the avocado pesto and serve.

34. BROCCOLI AND TOMATOES AIR FRIED STEW

Ready in about: 30 min | **Servings:** 4

INGREDIENTS:

- 2 tsp. coriander seeds
- 1 broccoli head, florets separated
- 1 tbsp. olive oil
- salt and black pepper to taste
- 1 yellow onion, chopped
- 28 ounces canned tomatoes, pureed
- 1 pinch of red pepper, crushed
- 1 garlic clove, minced
- 1 small ginger piece, chopped

DIRECTIONS:

Heat a pan suitable for your air fryer with oil over medium heat, add the onion, salt, pepper and chili, stir and cook for 7 minutes. Add ginger, garlic, coriander seeds, tomatoes, and broccoli, mix, place in the air fryer and cook at 360°F for 12 minutes. Divide into bowls and serve.

35. BROCCOLI MIX

Ready in about: 12 min | **Servings:** 2

INGREDIENTS:

- 2 cups vegetable broth
- 3 cups broccoli
- 1 tbsp. cumin powder
- 1 tbsp. cayenne powder
- 3 green onion
- salt to taste

DIRECTIONS:

Add vegetable broth into the air fryer pot. Combine broccoli, cumin powder, cayenne pepper powder, green onion and salt. Bake at 300°F for 20 minutes. When it's ready, serve.

36. BRUSSELS SPROUTS AND TOMATOES MIX

Ready in about: 15 min | **Servings:** 2

INGREDIENTS:

salt and black pepper
1-pound Brussels sprouts, trimmed

6 cherry tomatoes, halved
1 tbsp. olive oil

¼ cup green onions, chopped

DIRECTIONS:

Spice the Brussels sprouts with salt and pepper, put them in the air fryer and bake at 350°F for 10 minutes. Transfer them to a bowl, add salt, pepper, cherry tomatoes, onions greens, and olive oil, mix well and serve.

37. CHINESE BOWLS

Ready in about: 25 min | **Servings:** 4

INGREDIENTS:

3 tbsp. maple syrup
12 ounces firm tofu, cubed
¼ cup coconut aminos
2 tbsp. lime juice

2 tbsp. sesame oil
2 cup red quinoa, cooked
1-pound fresh Romanesco, roughly chopped

1 red bell pepper, chopped
3 carrots, chopped
8 ounces spinach, torn

DIRECTIONS:

In a bowl, mix the tofu cubes with oil, maple syrup, coconut aminos, and lime juice. Transfer into your air fryer and cook at 370°F for 15 minutes, stirring frequently. Add the romanesco, carrot, spinach, pepper, and quinoa. Divide into bowls and serve.

38. CHINESE CAULIFLOWER RICE

Ready in about: 30 min | **Servings:** 4

INGREDIENTS:

½ block firm tofu, cubed
4 tbsp. coconut aminos
1 cup carrot, chopped
1 tsp. turmeric powder

½ cup yellow onion, chopped
3 cups cauliflower, riced
1 tbsp. rice vinegar
1½ tsp. sesame oil

½ cup peas
½ cup broccoli florets, chopped
2 garlic cloves, minced
1 tbsp. ginger, minced

DIRECTIONS:

In a bowl, combine 2 tbsp. of tofu with coconut aminos, ½ cup onion, turmeric, and carrot. Mix to cover, transfer to the air fryer and cook at 370°F for 10 min, stirring halfway through cooking. Combine the cauliflower with the rest of the coconut aminos, sesame oil, garlic, vinegar, ginger, broccoli and peas. Stir, add the tofu mixture from the fryer, mix and cook everything at 370°F for 10 min. Divide between plates and serve.

39. CHINESE LONG BEANS MIX

Ready in about: 20 min | **Servings:** 3

INGREDIENTS:

- 1 tbsp. olive oil
- ½ tsp. coconut aminos
- 1 pinch of salt and black pepper
- 4 long beans, trimmed and sliced
- 4 garlic cloves, minced

DIRECTIONS:

In a pan suitable for your air fryer, combine the long beans with oil, coconut aminos, salt, pepper, and garlic, mix, place in your air fryer and cook at 350°F for 10 minutes. Divide between plates and serve.

40. COLLARD GREENS AND TOMATOES

Ready in about: 20 min | **Servings:** 4

INGREDIENTS:

- ¼ cup cherry tomatoes, halved
- 1-pound collard greens
- 1 tbsp. apple cider vinegar
- salt and black pepper to taste
- 2 tbsp. veggie stock

DIRECTIONS:

In a pan suitable for your air fryer, combine the tomatoes, collard greens, vinegar, broth, salt, and pepper, mix, place in the air fryer and cook at 320°F for 10 minutes. Divide between plates and serve.

41. COLLARD GREENS MIX

Ready in about: 20 min | **Servings:** 4

INGREDIENTS:

- 2 tbsp. olive oil
- 1 bunch collard greens, trimmed
- 2 tbsp. tomato puree
- 3 garlic cloves, minced
- 1 yellow onion, chopped
- salt and black pepper to taste
- 1 tsp. sugar
- 1 tbsp. balsamic vinegar

DIRECTIONS:

In a dish suitable for your air fryer, combine the oil, garlic, vinegar, onion and tomato puree and whisk. Add the cabbage, salt, pepper and sugar, mix, place in the fryer and cook at 320°F for 10 minutes. Divide the collard greens among plates and serve.

42. COOL TOFU MIX

Ready in about: 20 min │ **Servings:** 4

INGREDIENTS:

1 cup kale, torn
3 ounces firm tofu, pressed and crumbled
½ cup broccoli florets
¼ cup cherry tomatoes, halved

½ cup mushrooms, halved
½ cup carrot, grated
¼ tsp. onion powder
¼ cup microgreens
¼ tsp. garlic powder
½ tsp. yellow curry powder

salt and black pepper to taste
¼ tsp. sweet paprika
vegan cooking spray

DIRECTIONS:

Heat up your air fryer to 380°F, grease the pan with cooking spray, add the tofu, kale, broccoli, mushrooms, tomatoes, carrots, garlic powder, onion powder, paprika, salt, and pepper, mix, cover, and cook 10 minutes. Divide between plates, add the micro vegetables, mix and serve.

43. CORIANDER ENDIVES

Ready in about: 20 min │ **Servings:** 4

INGREDIENTS:

1 tbsp. coriander, chopped
2 endives, trimmed and halved

1 tsp. sweet paprika
1 pinch of salt and black pepper

½ cup almonds, chopped
2 tbsp. olive oil
2 tbsp. white vinegar

DIRECTIONS:

Toss the endive with cilantro and other ingredients in the air fryer's pan, mix, bake at 350°F for 15 minutes, divided into dishes and serve.

44. CORN SALAD

Ready in about: 20 min │ **Servings:** 2

INGREDIENTS:

1 drizzle of olive oil
3 cups corn
salt and black pepper
1 tbsp. stevia
1 tsp. sweet paprika

½ tsp. garlic powder
1 romaine lettuce head, cut into medium strip
12 cherry tomatoes, sliced

1 cup canned black beans, drained
4 green onions, chopped
3 tbsp. cilantro, chopped

DIRECTIONS:

Place the corn in a pan suitable for your air fryer, add a drizzle of oil, add salt, pepper, paprika, stevia and garlic powder, put it in the air fryer and cook at 350°F for 10 min. Transfer the corn to a salad bowl, add the lettuce, black beans, tomatoes, green onions, and cilantro, toss, divide and serve.

45. GARLIC EGGPLANTS

Ready in about: 20 min | **Servings:** 4

INGREDIENTS:

- 2 garlic cloves, minced
- 2 tbsp. olive oil
- 3 eggplants, halved and sliced
- 1 green onion stalk, chopped
- 1 red chili pepper, chopped
- 1 tbsp. ginger, grated
- 1 tbsp. balsamic vinegar
- 1 tbsp. coconut aminos

DIRECTIONS:

Heat a pan suitable for your air fryer with oil over medium-high heat, add the eggplant slices and cook for minutes. Add the chili, garlic, green onions, ginger, coconut aminos, and vinegar, place it in the air fryer and cook at 320°F for 7 minutes. Divide between plates and serve.

46. GREEN BEANS SALAD

Ready in about: 25 min | **Servings:** 4

INGREDIENTS:

- salt and black pepper to taste
- 1-pound green beans
- 1-pint cherry tomatoes
- 2 tbsp. olive oil

DIRECTIONS:

In a portable bowl, combine the cherry tomatoes with the green beans, olive oil, salt, and pepper, toss, transfer to a suitable pan for your air fryer and cook at 400°F for 15 minutes. Divide between plates and serve.

47. GREEN SALAD

Ready in about: 20 min | **Servings:** 4

INGREDIENTS:

- 4 red bell peppers
- 1 tbsp. lemon juice
- 1 lettuce head, cut into strips
- 1 ounce rocket leaves
- 3 tbsp. coconut cream
- salt and black pepper to taste
- 2 tbsp. olive oil

DIRECTIONS:

Spot the peppers in the basket of the air fryer, cook at 400°F for 10 minutes, transfer them to a bowl, let them cool on the side, peel them, cut them into strips and put them in a bowl. Add the arugula leaves and lettuce strips and mix. In a bowl, mix the oil with the lemon juice, coconut cream, salt, and pepper, beat well, add the salad, toss to coat, divide into plates and serve.

48. HOT CABBAGE MIX

Ready in about: 30 min | **Servings:** 2

INGREDIENTS:

- 1 yellow onion, chopped
- ½ cabbage head, chopped
- salt and black pepper to taste
- 1 dash of Tabasco sauce
- 1 cup coconut cream

DIRECTIONS:

Place the cabbage in a pan suitable for your air fryer. Add onion, salt, pepper, Tabasco sauce, and coconut cream, mix, put in the air fryer and cook at 400°F for 20 minutes. Divide between plates and serve.

49. INDIAN POTATOES

Ready in about: 22 min | **Servings:** 3

INGREDIENTS:

- 1 tbsp. cumin seeds
- 1 tbsp. coriander seeds
- salt and black pepper to taste
- ½ tsp. red chili powder
- ½ tsp. turmeric powder
- 1 tsp. pomegranate powder
- 2 tbsp. olive oil
- 2 tsp. fenugreek, dried
- 1 tbsp. pickled mango, chopped
- 5 potatoes, boiled, peeled, and cubed

DIRECTIONS:

Heat a pan suitable for your fryer with oil over medium heat, add the coriander and cumin seeds, stir and cook for 2 minutes. Add salt, pepper, turmeric, chili powder, pomegranate powder, mango, fenugreek, and potatoes, mix, place in an air fryer and cook at 360°F for 10 minutes. Divide among plates and serve hot.

50. KALE SANDWICH

Ready in about: 16 min | **Servings:** 1

INGREDIENTS:

- 2 cups kale, torn
- 1 drizzle of olive oil
- 1 pinch of salt and black pepper
- 1 small shallot, chopped
- 2 tbsp. pumpkin seeds
- ½ tsp. jalapeno, dried and crushed
- 1 vegan bun, halved
- 1 avocado slice
- 1½ tbsp. avocado mayonnaise

DIRECTIONS:

Heat your air fryer with oil to 360°F, add cabbage, salt, pepper, pumpkin seeds, green onions and jalapeño, mix, cover and cook for 6 minutes, shaking once. Spread the avocado mayonnaise on each half of the muffin, add the avocado slice, add the kale mixture, top with the other half of the muffin and serve.

51. LEEKS MEDLEY

Ready in about: 22 min | **Servings:** 4

INGREDIENTS:

1 tbsp. cumin, ground
6 leeks, roughly chopped
1 tbsp. mint, chopped

salt and black pepper to taste
1 tsp. garlic, minced

1 tbsp. parsley, chopped
1 drizzle of olive oil

DIRECTIONS:

In a pan suitable for your air fryer, mix the leeks with the cumin, mint, parsley, garlic, salt, pepper, and o
mix, place in your air fryer and cook at 350°F for 12 minutes. Divide the leek mixture between plates and serv

52. MEDITERRANEAN CHICKPEAS

Ready in about: 22 min | **Servings:** 2

INGREDIENTS:

3 shallots, chopped
vegan cooking spray
2 garlic cloves, minced
½ tsp. smoked paprika

½ tsp. sweet paprika
1 tbsp. parsley, chopped
½ tsp. cinnamon powder
2 tomatoes, chopped

salt and black pepper to taste
2 cup chickpeas, cooked

DIRECTIONS:

Spray the air fryer with cooking spray and preheat to 365°F. Add the shallots, garlic, smoked paprik
cinnamon, salt, pepper, tomatoes, parsley, and chickpeas, mix, cover and cook for 12 min. Divide and serve.

53. MEXICAN PEPPERS MIX

Ready in about: 28 min | **Servings:** 4

INGREDIENTS:

½ cup tomato juice
4 bell peppers, cutted
2 tbsp. jalapenos, chopped
¼ cup yellow onion, chopped

1 cup tomatoes, chopped
¼ cup green peppers, chopped
2 tsp. onion powder
1 tsp. cumin, ground

1 tsp. chili powder
½ tsp. red pepper, crushed
½ tsp. garlic powder
salt and black pepper to taste

DIRECTIONS:

In a pan suitable for your air fryer, combine the tomato juice, jalapeño, tomatoes, onion, green peppers, s
pepper, onion powder, red pepper, chili powder, garlic powder, cumin. Mix well in your air fryer and cook
350°F for 6 min Add the peppers and cook at 320°F for another 10 min. Divide the pepper mixture betwe
plates and serve.

54. OKRA AND CORN SALAD

Ready in about: 22 min | **Servings:** 6

INGREDIENTS:

6 scallions, chopped
1-pound okra, trimmed
3 green bell peppers, chopped

2 tbsp. olive oil
salt and black pepper to taste
1 tsp. sugar

28 ounces canned tomatoes, chopped

DIRECTIONS:

Warmth up a pan that fits your air fryer with the oil over medium-high heat, add the scallions and peppers, stir and cook for 5 minutes. Add okra, salt, pepper, sugar, tomatoes, and corn, mix, place in air fryer and cook at 30°F for 7 minutes. Divide the okra mixture between plates and serve hot.

55. ONION AND TOFU MIX

Ready in about: 25 min | **Servings:** 2

INGREDIENTS:

1 yellow onion, sliced
2 tbsp. flax meal mixed with 3 tbsp. water

1 tsp. coconut aminos
¼ cup firm tofu, cubed
1 pinch of black pepper

vegan cooking spray

DIRECTIONS:

In a bowl, mix flax flour with coconut aminos and the pepper black and mix well. Grease your air fryer with cooking spray, preheat to 350°F, add onion slices and cook for 10 minutes. Add the flax flour and the tofu, cook for another 5 minutes, divide into 2 plates and serve.

56. OREGANO BELL PEPPERS

Ready in about: 25 min | **Servings:** 4

INGREDIENTS:

1 sweet onion, chopped
1 tbsp. olive oil
1 red bell pepper, chopped

1 green bell pepper, chopped
1 orange bell pepper, chopped
salt and black pepper to taste

1 tbsp. oregano, chopped
½ cup cashew cheese, shredded

DIRECTIONS:

In a pan suitable for your air fryer, mix the onion with the red pepper, green pepper, orange pepper, salt, pepper, oregano and oil, mix, place in the air fryer and cook at 320°F for 10 minutes. Add the cashews, mix, place in the air fryer for another 4 minutes, divide between your plates and serve.

57. PAPRIKA BROCCOLI

Ready in about: 30 min | **Servings:** 4

INGREDIENTS:

juice of ½ lemon

1 broccoli head, florets separated

1 tbsp. olive oil

1 tbsp. sesame seeds

salt and black pepper to taste

2 tsp. paprika

3 garlic cloves, minced

DIRECTIONS:

In a portable bowl, toss the broccoli with the lemon juice, oil, paprika, salt, pepper and garlic and toss to co. Transfer in the basket of the air fryer, bake at 360°F for 15 minutes, sprinkle sesame seeds, cook another minutes, divide between the plates and serve.

58. PUMPKIN TASTY SEEDS

Ready in about: 16 min | **Servings:** 3

INGREDIENTS:

2 tbsp. olive oil

1 onion, chopped

1 carrot, chopped

2 cloves garlic, minced

2 tsp. curry powder

salt to taste

4 cups vegetable broth

2 tbsp. pumpkin seeds

parsley to garnish

DIRECTIONS:

Add oil into the air fryer pot. Combine the onion, carrots, garlic, curry powder, vegetable broth, pumpkin see and salt. Bake at 300°F for 15 minutes. When it's ready, garnish with the parsley to serve.

59. RED POTATOES AND GREEN BEANS

Ready in about: 25 min | **Servings:** 4

INGREDIENTS:

1-pound green beans

1-pound red potatoes, cut into wedges

2 garlic cloves, minced

½ tsp. oregano, dried

salt and black pepper to taste

2 tbsp. olive oil

DIRECTIONS:

In a pan suitable for your air fryer, mix the potatoes with the green beans, garlic, oil, salt, pepper, and orega mix, place in your air fryer and cook at 380°F for 15 minutes. Divide between plates and serve.

60. RICE AND VEGGIES

Ready in about: 20 min | **Servings:** 4

INGREDIENTS:

1 tbsp. olive oil
2 cups rice, cooked

salt and black pepper to taste
2 carrots, chopped

10 tbsp. coconut cream
4 garlic cloves, minced
3 small broccoli florets

DIRECTIONS:

Warm your air fryer to 350°F, add the oil, garlic, carrots, broccoli, salt, and pepper and mix. Add the rice and coconut cream, mix, cover and cook for 10 minutes. Divide the rice and vegetables between plates and serve.

61. RICE MIXED BEANS

Ready in about: 15 min | **Servings:** 3

INGREDIENTS:

1 onion, diced
2 garlic cloves
2 cups brown rice, boiled

2 cups black beans
2 cups water
salt to taste

1 avocado, cubes

DIRECTIONS:

Add onion into the air fryer pot. Combine the garlic, brown rice, black beans, water, avocado, and salt. Cook at 350°F for 20 minutes. When it's ready, serve!

62. SCRAMBLED TOFU

Ready in about: 40 min | **Servings:** 4

INGREDIENTS:

1 block firm tofu, cubed
2 tbsp. coconut aminos
1 tsp. turmeric powder
½ tsp. onion powder

salt and black pepper to taste
2 tbsp. olive oil
½ tsp. garlic powder

½ cup yellow onion, chopped
2½ cup red potatoes, cubed

DIRECTIONS:

In a bowl, combine the tofu with 1 tbsp. of oil, salt, pepper, coconut aminos, powdered garlic and onion, turmeric and onion and toss to coat. In another bowl, toss the potatoes with the remaining oil, salt and pepper and toss. Place the potatoes in an air fryer preheated to 350°F and bake in oven for 15 minutes shaking in two. Add the tofu and marinade and bake at 350°F for 15 minutes. Divide into plates and serve.

63. SUMMER SQUASH MIX

Ready in about: 20 min | **Servings:** 4

INGREDIENTS:

- ½ tsp. oregano, dried
- 3 ounces coconut cream
- salt and black pepper to taste
- ⅓ cup carrot, cubed
- 1 big yellow summer squash, peeled and cubed
- 2 tbsp. olive oil

DIRECTIONS:

In a pan suitable for your air fryer, mix the squash with the carrot, oil, oregano, salt, pepper, and cocon cream, mix, transfer to the air fryer and cook at 400°F for 10 minutes. Divide between plates and serve.

64. TOFU CASSEROLE

Ready in about: 30 min | **Servings:** 4

INGREDIENTS:

- 14 ounces tofu, cubed
- 1 tsp. lemon zest, grated
- 1 tbsp. lemon juice
- 1 tbsp. apple cider vinegar
- 2 tbsp. nutritional yeast
- 1 tbsp. olive oil
- 10 ounces spinach, torn
- 2 garlic cloves, minced
- ½ cup yellow onion, chopped
- 8 ounces mushrooms, sliced
- vegan cooking spray
- ½ tsp. basil, dried
- ¼ tsp. red pepper flakes
- salt and black pepper to taste

DIRECTIONS:

Spray your air fryer with cooking spray, place the tofu cubes background in, add the lemon zest, lemon jui yeast, vinegar, oil of olive, garlic, spinach, the onion, basil, mushrooms, salt, and pepper; mix, cover, and ba at 365°F for 20 minutes. Divide among plates and serve.

65. TOMATO FRITTATA

Ready in about: 40 min | **Servings:** 2

INGREDIENTS:

- ½ cup cashew cheese, shredded
- 2 tbsp. flax meal mixed with 3 tbsp. water
- 2 tbsp. yellow onion, chopped
- ¼ cup tomatoes, chopped
- ¼ cup coconut milk
- salt and black pepper to taste

DIRECTIONS:

In a bowl, mix the flax flour with the milk, cheese, salt, pepper, onion, and tomatoes, mix well, pour into pan of your air fryer, cover and cook at 340°F for 30 minutes. Divide the omelet between plates and serve.

66. TOMATOES AND BELL PEPPERS MIX

eady in about: 25 min | **Servings:** 4

GREDIENTS:

- 2 garlic cloves, minced
- 2 red bell peppers, chopped
- 1-pound cherry tomatoes, halved
- 3 bay leaves
- 1 tsp. rosemary, dried
- 2 tbsp. olive oil
- salt and black pepper to taste
- 1 tbsp. balsamic vinegar

RECTIONS:

an enormous bowl, combine the tomatoes with the garlic, salt, black pepper, rosemary, bay leaves, half the and half the vinegar, toss to cover, place in your air fryer and roast at 320°F. for 15 minutes. In your food ocessor, mix the peppers with salt, the black pepper, the rest of the oil, and the remaining vinegar and mix ll. Divide the roasted tomatoes between the plates, pour in the pepper sauce and serve.

67. TURNIPS SIDE SALAD

eady in about: 20 min | **Servings:** 4

GREDIENTS:

- 1 tsp. garlic, minced
- 20 ounces turnips, peeled and chopped
- 1 tsp. ginger, grated
- 2 tomatoes, chopped
- 2 yellow onions, chopped
- 1 tsp. cumin, ground
- 2 green chilies, chopped
- 1 tsp. coriander, ground
- ½ tsp. turmeric powder
- salt and black pepper to taste
- 1 tbsp. olive oil

RECTIONS:

armth up a pan that fits your air fryer with oil over medium-high heat, add green peppers, garlic, and ginger, r and cook for 1 minute. Add onions, salt, pepper, tomatoes, turmeric, cumin, the coriander ground, and nips, mix, place in the air fryer and bake at 350°F for 10 minutes. Divide between plates and serve.

68. VEGETABLE BROTH WITH VEGGIES SOUP

ady in about: 20 min | **Servings:** 3

GREDIENTS:

- 2 tbsp. olive oil
- 1 onion, chopped
- 2 cups vegetable broth
- 3 potatoes, diced
- 1 tsp. thyme
- 2 tbsp. apple cider vinegar
- 2 carrots, sliced
- parsley to garnish

RECTIONS:

d oil into the air fryer pot. Combine onion, vegetable stock, potatoes, thyme, apple vinegar, and carrots.)k at 300°F for 15 minutes. When it's ready, garnish with the parsley to serve.

69. VEGGIE BROTH WITH CAULIFLOWER

Ready in about: 16 min | **Servings:** 2

INGREDIENTS:

- 2 carrots, sliced
- 2 cups vegetable broth
- salt to taste
- 4 cups cauliflower florets
- 2 tbsp. garlic, minced
- 2 tbsp. thyme, dried
- 4 celery stalks
- 1 tbsp. cornstarch

DIRECTIONS:

Add vegetable broth into the air fryer pot. Mix carrot, cauliflower, garlic, thyme, celery stems, cornstarch, and salt. Cook at 300°F for 20 minutes. Serve and enjoy!

70. VEGGIE CASSEROLE

Ready in about: 25 min | **Servings:** 4

INGREDIENTS:

- ¾ cup cashews, soaked for 30 minutes and drained
- 2 tsp. onion powder
- ¼ cup nutritional yeast
- ½ tsp. sage, dried
- 1 tsp. garlic powder
- salt and black pepper to taste
- ½ cup cilantro, chopped
- 2 tsp. olive oil
- 1½ cup spinach, chopped
- ¾ cup red onion, chopped
- 4 garlic cloves, minced

DIRECTIONS:

In a pan suitable for your air fryer, mix the lentils with the chili, ginger, turmeric, garam masala, salt, pepper, olive oil, cilantro, spinach, onion, and garlic, stir, place in your air fryer and cook at 400°F for 15 minutes. Divide the lentil mixture between plates and serve.

71. WHITE MUSHROOMS MIX

Ready in about: 25 min | **Servings:** 2

INGREDIENTS:

- 7 ounces snow peas
- salt and black pepper to taste
- 8 ounces white mushrooms, halved
- 1 tsp. olive oil
- 2 tbsp. coconut aminos
- 1 yellow onion, cut into rings

DIRECTIONS:

In a portable bowl, peas with mushrooms, onion, coconut aminos, oil, salt, and pepper, mix well, transfer to a saucepan suitable for your air fryer, place in the air fryer and cook at 350°F for 15 minutes. Divide between plates and serve.

72. YAM MIX

Ready in about: 18 min | **Servings:** 4

INGREDIENTS:

- ½ tsp. cinnamon powder
- 16 ounces canned candied yams, drained
- ¼ tsp. allspice, ground
- 1 tbsp. flax meal mixed with 2 tbsp. water
- ½ cup coconut sugar
- 2 tbsp. coconut cream
- vegan cooking spray
- ½ cup maple syrup

DIRECTIONS:

In a bowl, combine the sweet potatoes with the cinnamon and all the spices, mash with a fork and mix well. Grease your air fryer with cooking spray, preheat to 400°F. Add the sweet potato mixture to the bottom. Add the sugar, flax flour, coconut cream, and maple syrup, mix gently, cover and cook for 8 min. Serve.

73. ZUCCHINI AND SQUASH SALAD

Ready in about: 35 min | **Servings:** 4

INGREDIENTS:

- 1-pound zucchinis, cut into half moons
- 6 tsp. olive oil
- ½ pound carrots, cubed
- salt and white pepper to taste
- 2 tbsp. tomato paste
- 1 yellow squash, cut into chunks
- 1 tbsp. tarragon, chopped

DIRECTIONS:

In your air fryer's pan, mix oil with zucchinis, carrots, squash, salt, pepper, tarragon, and tomato paste, cover and cook at 400°F for 25 minutes. Divide between plates and serve.

74. ZUCCHINI AND SWEET POTATOES

Ready in about: 25 min | **Servings:** 8

INGREDIENTS:

- 2 tbsp. olive oil
- 1 cup veggie stock
- salt and pepper
- 2 sweet potatoes, peeled and cutted
- 2 yellow onions, chopped
- 8 zucchinis, cutted
- 1 cup coconut milk
- 1 tbsp. coconut aminos

DIRECTIONS:

Warm up a pan that fits your air fryer with the oil over medium heat, add onion, stir and cook for 2 min. Add zucchinis, potato, salt, pepper, stock, milk, aminos, and dill, stir, introduce in your air fryer, cook at 360°F for min, divide between plates and serve.

SIDE DISHES

"Animal protection isn't a radical idea.
It follows the simple principle that if animals feel pain, joy and fear,
they should be protected from suffering."

— Anonymous

75. AIR FRIED ROSEMARY CHIPS

Ready in about: 60 min | **Servings:** 4

INGREDIENTS:

- 4 russet potatoes
- ¼ tsp. of salt
- 2 tsp. of finely chopped rosemary
- 3 tsp. of olive oil

DIRECTIONS:

Peel the potatoes and cut them into thin slices. Soak in water for approximately 30 minutes, drain, then d
with paper towels. Heat your air fryer to about 330°F. Pour the olive oil on the chips and stir until all potato
are coated. Spot the potatoes in the air fryer basket and fry them for 30 minutes until golden and crispy. M
frequently during the cooking to ensure that the potatoes cook evenly. Remove from the fryer, add the rosema
and salt and toss to combine.

76. ARABIC PLUMS MIX

Ready in about: 22 min | **Servings:** 4

INGREDIENTS:

- 3 ounces almonds, peeled and chopped
- 3 tbsp. stevia
- 12 ounces plumps, pitted
- 2 yellow onions, chopped
- 2 tbsp. veggie stock
- 2 garlic cloves, minced
- 1 tsp. cumin powder
- salt and black pepper to taste
- 3 tbsp. olive oil
- 1 tsp. turmeric powder
- 1 tsp. cinnamon powder
- 1 tsp. ginger powder

DIRECTIONS:

In a saucepan suitable for your air fryer, combine the almonds with the plums, stevia, broth, onion, garlic, s
pepper, cumin, turmeric, ginger, cinnamon, and oil, mix, place in your air fryer and cook at 350°F for
minutes. Divide the plum mixture between the dishes and serve.

77. BABY CARROTS

Ready in about: 22 min | **Servings:** 4

INGREDIENTS:

- salt and black pepper taste
- 1 tbsp. olive oil
- 3 cups baby carrots
- 1 tbsp. stevia

DIRECTIONS:

In a portable bowl, toss the carrots with salt, pepper, oil, and stevia, toss to coat, transfer the carrots to the
fryer and cook at 400°F for 12 minutes. Divide them between plates and serve.

78. BABY CARROTS AND PARSLEY

Ready in about: 20 min | **Servings:** 4

INGREDIENTS:

salt and black pepper to taste

½ tbsp. olive oil

2 cups baby carrots

1 tbsp. parsley, chopped

DIRECTIONS:

In a saucepan that matches your air fryer, the carrots mixed with oil, pepper, and parsley, turning, introduces your air fryer and cook at 350°F for 10 minutes. Divide between the plates and serve.

79. BABY POTATOES SALAD

Ready in about: 30 min | **Servings:** 4

INGREDIENTS:

2 garlic cloves, chopped

1½ pounds baby potatoes, halved

2 red onions, chopped

3 tbsp. olive oil

9 ounces cherry tomatoes

1½ tbsp. balsamic vinegar

salt and black pepper to taste

2 thyme springs, chopped

DIRECTIONS:

In your food processor, mix the garlic with the onion, oil, vinegar, thyme, salt, and pepper and mix very well. In a portable bowl, mix the potatoes with the tomatoes and the balsamic mixture, mix, put in the air fryer and cook at 380°F for 20 minutes. Divide among plates and serve cold.

80. BALSAMIC ARTICHOKES

Ready in about: 17 min | **Servings:** 4

INGREDIENTS:

salt and black pepper to taste

4 big artichokes, trimmed

2 tbsp. lemon juice

2 tsp. balsamic vinegar

2 garlic cloves, minced

¼ cup extra virgin olive oil

1 tsp. oregano, dried

DIRECTIONS:

Season the artichokes with salt and pepper, rub them with half the oil and half the lemon juice, put them in your air fryer and cook at 360°F for 7 minutes. Meanwhile, in a bowl, combine the remaining lemon juice with the vinegar, remaining oil, salt, pepper, garlic, and oregano and mix well. Arrange the artichokes on a serving platter, sprinkle with balsamic vinaigrette and serve.

81. BEET SALAD AND PARSLEY DRESSING

Ready in about: 24 min | **Servings:** 4

INGREDIENTS:

- 4 beets
- 1 bunch of parsley, chopped
- 2 tbsp. balsamic vinegar
- salt and black pepper to taste
- 2 tbsp. capers
- 1 garlic clove, chopped
- 1 tbsp. extra virgin olive oi

DIRECTIONS:

Place the beets in your air fryer and cook them at 360°F for 14 min. Meanwhile, in a bowl, combine the parsle garlic, salt, pepper, the oil of olive and capers and mix well. Transfer the beets to a cutting board, let them coc peel them, slice them and put them in a salad bowl. Add vinegar, drizzle with parsley vinaigrette and serve.

82. BEET SIDE SALAD

Ready in about: 24 min | **Servings:** 4

INGREDIENTS:

- 2 tbsp. balsamic vinegar
- 4 beets, trimmed
- 1 bunch of parsley, chopped
- 2 tbsp. capers
- 1 tbsp. extra-virgin olive oil
- salt and black pepper to taste
- 1 garlic clove, chopped

DIRECTIONS:

Place the beets in the basket of your air fryer and cook them at 360°F for 14 minutes. In a bowl, combine t parsley with the garlic, salt, pepper, olive oil, and capers and mix well. Leave the beets to cool, peel them, c them into slices, put them in a bowl, add the vinegar and parsley, mix, distribute among plates and serve.

83. BEETS AND ARUGULA SALAD

Ready in about: 20 min | **Servings:** 4

INGREDIENTS:

- 1 drizzle of olive oil
- 1½ pounds beets, peeled
- 2 tsp. orange zest, grated
- ½ cup orange juice
- 2 tbsp. cider vinegar
- 2 cups arugula
- 2 tbsp. brown sugar
- 2 tsp. mustard
- 2 scallions, chopped

DIRECTIONS:

Rub beets with the oil and orange juice, put them in the air fryer and bake at 350°F for 10 minutes. Trans the beetroot wedges to a bowl, add the shallots, arugula, and the zest of orange and mix. In another bo combine the sugar with the mustard and vinegar, mix well, add to the salad, toss and serve.

84. BELL PEPPERS

Ready in about: 20 min | **Servings:** 8

INGREDIENTS:

- 1 orange bell pepper, halved
- 1 yellow bell pepper, halved
- salt and black pepper to taste
- 1 green onion, chopped
- 3½ ounces firm tofu, crumbled
- 2 tbsp. oregano, chopped

DIRECTIONS:

In a bowl, combine the tofu with the onion, salt, pepper and oregano and mix well. Place the pepper halves in the basket of your air fryer and bake at 400°F for 10 minutes. Let the bell pepper halves cool, peel, spread the tofu mixture over each piece, roll up, arrange on plates and serve immediately.

85. BORLOTTI BEANS WITH TOMATO SAUCE

Ready in about: 16 min | **Servings:** 3

INGREDIENTS:

- 2 tbsp. oregano powder
- 2 cups tomato sauce
- 1 tbsp. red pepper flakes
- 2 tbsp. oil
- 1 carrot, sliced
- salt to taste
- 2 garlic cloves
- 2 cups Borlotti beans
- 1 onion, chopped

DIRECTIONS:

Add oil into the air fryer pot. Add the tomato sauce, oregano powder, red pepper flakes, carrot, garlic, onion, salt and borlotti beans. Cook at 300°F for 20 minutes. Serve and enjoy!

86. BROCCOLI AND ALMONDS

Ready in about: 17 min | **Servings:** 4

INGREDIENTS:

- ½ cup almonds; chopped
- 1 lb. broccoli florets
- 3 garlic cloves; minced
- 1 pinch of salt and black pepper
- 2 tbsp. red vinegar
- 1 tbsp. chives; chopped
- 3 tbsp. coconut oil; melted

DIRECTIONS:

Take a bowl and mix the broccoli with the garlic, salt, pepper, vinegar, and oil and mix. Place the broccoli in the basket of the air fryer and cook for 12 minutes at 350°F. Divide between plates and serve with a pinch of almonds and chives.

87. BRUSSELS SPROUTS AND POMEGRANATE SEEDS

Ready in about: 15 min | **Servings:** 4

INGREDIENTS:

- salt and black pepper to taste
- 1-pound Brussels sprouts, trimmed and halved
- 1 cup pomegranate seeds
- 2 tbsp. veggie stock
- 1 tbsp. olive oil
- ¼ cup pine nuts, toasted

DIRECTIONS:

In a heat-resistant dish suitable for your air fryer, mix the Brussels sprouts with salt, pepper, pomegranate seeds, pine nuts, oil and broth, mix, place in your basket of air fryer and cook at 390°F times 10 minutes. Divide between plates and serve.

88. BRUSSELS SPROUTS MIX

Ready in about: 40 min | **Servings:** 8

INGREDIENTS:

- 1 drizzle of olive oil
- 3 pounds Brussels sprouts, halved
- 4 shallots, chopped
- salt and black pepper to taste
- 4 tbsp. whole wheat flour
- 1 tbsp. thyme, chopped
- 1 cup coconut cream
- ¼ tsp. nutmeg, ground
- 4 tbsp. horseradish

DIRECTIONS:

In a portable bowl, combine the sprouts with a little oil, salt, and pepper, toss to coat, place in the air fryer, cook at 400°F for 20 minutes and transfer to a pan that fits your fryer. Add the shallot, flour mixed with coconut cream, nutmeg, and thyme, mix, put the pan in the air fryer and cook at 400°F for another 10 minutes. Divide the sprouts between plates, garnish with horseradish and serve.

89. CAJUN ONION MIX

eady in about: 2 h 15 min | **Servings:** 4

IGREDIENTS:

- salt and black pepper
- 2 big white onions, cut into medium chunks
- ¼ cup coconut cream
- 1½ tsp. paprika
- ½ tsp. Cajun seasoning
- 1 drizzle of olive oil
- 1 tsp. garlic powder1

IRECTIONS:

a a pan suitable for your air fryer, mix the onion pieces with salt, pepper, cream, oil, paprika, garlic powder, d Cajun seasoning, stir, place the pan in your air fryer and cook at 360°F for 15 minutes. Divide the onion ixture between plates and serve.

90. CARROTS AND RHUBARB

eady in about: 50 min | **Servings:** 4

GREDIENTS:

- 2 tsp. walnut oil
- 1-pound baby carrots
- 1-pound rhubarb, roughly chopped
- ½ tsp. stevia
- ½ cup walnuts, halved
- 1 orange, peeled, cut into medium segments and zest grated

IRECTIONS:

t the oil in your air fryer, add the carrots, mix them together and fry them at 380°F for 20 minutes. Add the ubarb, orange zest, stevia, and walnuts, mix and cook for another 20 minutes. Add the orange slices, toss d serve.

91. CARROT MIX

eady in about: 25 min | **Servings:** 4

GREDIENTS:

- ½ cup steel cut oats
- 2 cups coconut milk
- 1 cup carrots, shredded
- 1 tsp. cardamom, ground
- 1 pinch of saffron
- ½ tsp. agave nectar
- vegan cooking spray

IRECTIONS:

ray your air fryer with cooking spray, add milk, oatmeal, carrots, cardamom, and agave nectar, mix, cover l cook at 365°F for 15 minutes. Divide into bowls, sprinkle with saffron and serve

92. CHICKPEAS FALAFEL WITH YOGURT SAUCE

Ready in about: 20 min | **Servings:** 4

INGREDIENTS:

- 1 can chickpeas, rinsed, drained, and dried
- 1 small yellow onion, quartered
- 3 cloves garlic, roughly chopped
- ⅓ cup roughly chopped parsley
- ⅓ cup roughly chopped cilantro
- ⅓ cup chopped scallions
- 1 teaspoon cumin

- ½ tsp. kosher salt
- ⅛ tsp. crushed red pepper flakes
- 1 tsp. baking powder
- 4 tbsp all-purpose flour

For the sauce:
- 2 tbsp. lemon juice
- 1 clove garlic, grated or very finely minced
- 1 cup unsweetened Greek-styl vegan yogurt
- 3 tbsp. tahini paste
- 1 tsp. fine salt
- 5 tsp. olive oil

DIRECTIONS:

Place onion and garlic in a food processor. Add parsley, cilantro, scallions, cumin, red pepper flakes, and sa Process for one minute. Add the chickpeas and process them until just blended, then add the flour and t baking powder. Process for 5 seconds, then refrigerate, covered, 2 hours. Preheat the air fryer to 350°F, for the mixture into 12 balls and spry them with oil. Cook 14 minutes turning halfway. Serve.

For the sauce: in a bowl combine the garlic and lemon juice. Whisk in the yogurt, tahini, and salt. Store the fridge for up to 5 days.

93. CREAMY BRUSSELS SPROUTS

Ready in about: 15 min | **Servings:** 4

INGREDIENTS:

- salt and black pepper to taste

- 1-pound Brussels sprouts, trimmed
- 1 tbsp. mustard

- 2 tbsp. dill, chopped
- 2 tbsp. coconut cream

DIRECTIONS:

Place the Brussels sprouts in your air fryer basket and cook them at 350°F for 10 minutes. In a bowl, combi the cream with the mustard, dill, salt and pepper and mix. Add the Brussels sprouts, toss, divide between t plates and serve.

94. CREAMY POTATOES

Ready in about: 30 min | **Servings:** 8

INGREDIENTS:

2 pounds gold potatoes, halved and sliced

vegan cooking spray

1 yellow onion, cut into medium wedges

8 ounces coconut milk

10 ounces canned vegan potato cream soup

1 cup tofu, crumbled

salt and black pepper to taste

½ cup veggie stock

DIRECTIONS:

Grease your air fryer's pan with cooking spray and place half the potatoes on the bottom. Layer onion wedges, half of the vegan cream soup, coconut milk, tofu, stock, salt, and pepper. Add the rest of the potatoes, onion pieces, cream, coconut milk, tofu, and broth, cover and cook at 365°F for 20 minutes. Serve.

95. CRISPY POTATOES AND PARSLEY

Ready in about: 20 min | **Servings:** 4

INGREDIENTS:

salt and black pepper to taste

1-pound gold potatoes, cut into wedges

2 tbsp. olive

¼ cup parsley leaves, chopped

juice from ½ lemon

DIRECTIONS:

Rub the potatoes with salt, pepper, lemon juice, and olive oil, place them in the air fryer and bake at 350°F for minutes. Divide among plates, sprinkle with parsley and serve.

96. DELICIOUS CORN MIX

Ready in about: 52 min | **Servings:** 6

INGREDIENTS:

2 cups corn

1 tbsp. olive oil

1 yellow onion, chopped

½ cup red bell pepper, chopped

¼ cup celery, chopped

1 tsp. thyme, chopped

salt and black pepper to taste

2 tsp. garlic, minced

½ cup coconut cream

3 cups vegan breadcrumbs

1½ cups coconut milk

DIRECTIONS:

Heat a pan with oil over medium-high heat, add the corn, celery, onion, bell pepper, salt, pepper, garlic, and thyme, mix, cook 12 minutes and transfer to a pan suitable for your air fryer. Add the coconut milk, coconut cream and mix. Squeeze breadcrumbs over corn mixture, place in an air fryer and bake at 320°F for 40 minutes. Divide between plates and serve.

97. DELICIOUS POTATO MIX

Ready in about: 35 min | **Servings:** 6

INGREDIENTS:

3 garlic cloves, minced

6 ounces jarred roasted red bell peppers, chopped

2 tbsp. parsley, chopped

2 tbsp. chives, chopped

salt and black pepper to taste

vegan cooking spray

4 potatoes, peeled and cut into wedges

DIRECTIONS:

In a pan suitable for your air fryer, mix the roasted peppers with the garlic, parsley, salt, pepper, chives, pota wedges, and oil, mix, transfer to the air fryer and cook at 350°F for 25 minutes. Divide between plates a serve as a garnish.

98. DELICIOUS ROASTED CARROTS

Ready in about: 30 min | **Servings:** 4

INGREDIENTS:

2 tsp. olive oil

4 tbsp. orange juice

1-pound baby carrots

1 tsp. herbs de Provence

DIRECTIONS:

In your air fryer basket, combine the carrots with the Provence herbs, oil, and orange juice, mix and cook 320°F for 20 minutes. Divide between plates and serve as a garnish.

99. EASY PEPPERS

Ready in about: 35 min | **Servings:** 12

INGREDIENTS:

1 tbsp. olive oil

12 colored bell peppers, seedless and sliced

1 yellow onion, sliced

salt and black pepper to taste

½ tsp. smoked paprika

DIRECTIONS:

Put the oil in a pan suitable for your air fryer, add the peppers, paprika, and onion, mix, place the pan in yc air fryer and cook at 320°F for 25 minutes. Season with salt and pepper to taste, divide between dishes a serve.

100. EASY PORTOBELLO MUSHROOMS

Ready in about: 22 min | **Servings:** 4

INGREDIENTS:

1 tbsp. olive oil

4 big Portobello mushroom caps

1 cup spinach, torn

¼ tsp. rosemary, chopped

⅓ cup vegan breadcrumbs

DIRECTIONS:

Rub mushrooms caps with the oil, place them in the basket of the air fryer and cook at 350°F for 2 minutes. Meanwhile, in a bowl, combine the spinach, rosemary, and breadcrumbs and mix well. Fill the mushrooms with this mixture, put them in the air fryer basket and cook at 350°F for 10 minutes. Divide them between plates and serve.

101. EGGPLANT TASTY MIX

Ready in about: 20 min | **Servings:** 4

INGREDIENTS:

salt and black pepper to taste

8 baby eggplants, scooped in the center and pulp reserved

1 pinch of oregano, dried

1 tbsp. tomato paste

1 green bell pepper, chopped

1 bunch coriander, chopped

1 tbsp. olive oil

1 tomato chopped

½ tsp. garlic powder

1 yellow onion, chopped

DIRECTIONS:

Heat a portable pan with the oil over medium heat, add the onion, stir and cook for 1 minute. Add salt, pepper, eggplant pulp, oregano, green pepper, tomato paste, garlic powder, coriander, and tomato, mix, cook for 1-2 minutes, remove from heat and let cool. Add the eggplants to this mixture, place them in the basket of your air fryer and cook them at 360°F for 8 minutes. Divide eggplants between plates and serve them as a side dish.

102. FLAVORED CAULIFLOWER

Ready in about: 20 min | **Servings:** 4

INGREDIENTS:

- salt and black pepper to taste
- 12 cauliflower florets, steamed
- ¼ tsp. turmeric powder
- 1 tbsp. ginger, grated
- 1½ tsp. red chili powder
- 2 tsp. lemon juice
- 2 tbsp. water
- ½ tsp. corn flour
- 3 tbsp. white flour
- vegan cooking spray

DIRECTIONS:

In a bowl, mix the chili powder with the turmeric powder, ginger paste, salt, pepper, lemon juice, white flour, cornmeal, and water, mix, add cabbage - flower, mix well and transfer them to your air fryer basket. Coat with cooking spray, bake at 400°F for 10 minutes, divide into plates and serve as a garnish.

103. FRIED RED CABBAGE

Ready in about: 25 min | **Servings:** 4

INGREDIENTS:

- ½ cup yellow onion, chopped
- 4 garlic cloves, minced
- 1 tbsp. olive oil
- 1 cup veggie stock
- 6 cups red cabbage, chopped
- 1 tbsp. apple cider vinegar
- salt and black pepper to taste
- 1 cup applesauce

DIRECTIONS:

In a heat-resistant plate that fits your fryer, mix the cabbage with the onion, garlic, oil, broth, vinegar, applesauce, salt, and pepper, mix very well, put the dish in the basket of your air fryer and cook at 380°F for 15 minutes. Divide between plates and serve as a garnish.

104. GARLIC BEET WEDGES

Ready in about: 25 min | **Servings:** 4

INGREDIENTS:

- 1 tbsp. olive oil
- 4 beets, washed, peeled, and cut into large wedges
- salt and black to taste
- 1 tsp. lemon juice
- 2 garlic cloves, minced

DIRECTIONS:

In a bowl, combine the beets with the oil, salt, pepper, garlic, and lemon juice, mix well, transfer to your fryer basket and cook at 400°F for 15 minutes. Divide the beets wedges slices on plates and serve as a garni

105. GARLIC TOMATOES

Ready in about: 20 min | **Servings:** 4

INGREDIENTS:

6 garlic cloves; minced

1 lb. cherry tomatoes; halved

1 tbsp. olive oil

1 tbsp. balsamic vinegar

1 tbsp. dill; chopped.

salt and black pepper to taste

DIRECTIONS:

In a pan suitable for the air fryer, combine all the ingredients, mix gently. Place the pan in the air fryer and cook for 15 minutes at 380°F. Divide between plates and serve.

106. GLAZED BEETS

Ready in about: 60 min | **Servings:** 8

INGREDIENTS:

1 tbsp. olive oil

4 tbsp. maple syrup

3 pounds beetroots, peeled and cut into medium chunks

DIRECTIONS:

Rub the beets with oil, add the maple syrup, mix, put in the air fryer and cook at 350°F for 40 minutes. Divide between plates and serve.

107. GOLD POTATOES AND BELL PEPPER MIX

Ready in about: 35 min | **Servings:** 4

INGREDIENTS:

1 yellow onion, chopped

4 gold potatoes, cubed

2 tsp. olive oil

1 green bell pepper, chopped

½ tsp. thyme, dried

salt and black pepper to taste

DIRECTIONS:

Warmth up your air fryer to 350°F, add oil, heat it, add onion, pepper, salt and pepper, stir and cook for 5 minutes. Add the potatoes and thyme, mix, cover and cook at 360°F for 20 minutes. Divide between plates and serve.

108. GREEK POTATOES MIX

Ready in about: 30 min | **Servings:** 4

INGREDIENTS:

- 2 tbsp. olive oil
- 1½ pounds potatoes, peeled and cubed
- salt and black pepper to taste
- 3½ ounces coconut cream
- 1 tbsp. hot paprika

DIRECTIONS:

Put the potatoes in a bowl, add the water to cover, set aside for 10 minutes, drain, mix with half the oil, sa pepper and paprika and stir. Place the potatoes in your air fryer basket and cook at 360°F for 20 minutes. Ir bowl, combine the coconut cream with the salt, pepper, and the rest of the oil and mix well. Divide the potato between plates, add the coconut cream on top and serve.

109. GREEK VEGGIE

Ready in about: 55 min | **Servings:** 4

INGREDIENTS:

- 1 zucchini, sliced
- 1 eggplant, sliced
- 2 red bell peppers, chopped
- 3 tbsp. olive oil
- 2 garlic cloves, minced
- 1 bay leaf
- salt and black pepper to taste
- 2 onions, chopped
- 1 thyme spring, chopped
- 4 tomatoes, cut into quarters

DIRECTIONS:

In your pan, mix the eggplant slices with the zucchini slices, peppers, garlic, oil, bay leaf, thyme, onion, toma salt and pepper, mix and cook at 300°F for 35 minutes. Divide between plates and serve as a garnish.

110. GREEN BEANS

Ready in about: 35 min | **Servings:** 4

INGREDIENTS:

- salt and black pepper to taste
- 1½ pounds green beans, trimmed and steamed for 2 minutes
- ½ pound shallots, chopp
- 2 tbsp. olive oil
- ¼ cup almonds, toasted

DIRECTIONS:

In the air- fryer basket from the fryer, mix the beans with salt, pepper, chives, almonds, and oil, mix well a cook at 400°F for 25 minutes. Divide between plates and serve as a garnish.

111. HASSELBACK POTATOES

Ready in about: 30 min | **Servings:** 2

INGREDIENTS:

2 tbsp. olive oil

2 potatoes, peeled and thinly sliced almost all the way horizontally

1 tsp. garlic, minced

½ tsp. oregano, dried

½ tsp. sweet paprika

salt and black pepper to taste

½ tsp. basil, dried

DIRECTIONS:

In a bowl, combine the oil with the garlic, salt, pepper, oregano, basil, and paprika and mix well. Rub the potatoes with this mixture, put them in the basket of your air fryer and fry them for 20 minutes at 350°F. Divide them among plates and serve as a garnish.

112. HERBED EGGPLANT AND ZUCCHINI MIX

Ready in about: 18 min | **Servings:** 4

INGREDIENTS:

3 zucchinis, roughly cubed

1 eggplant, roughly cubed

2 tbsp. lemon juice

1 tsp. thyme, dried

3 tbsp. olive oil

salt and black pepper to taste

1 tsp. oregano, dried

DIRECTIONS:

Put the eggplant in a dish suitable for your air fryer, add the zucchini, the juice of lemon, salt, pepper, thyme, oregano and olive oil, mix, place the air fryer and cook at 360°F for 8 minutes. Divide between plates and serve immediately.

113. HERBED TOMATOES

Ready in about: 25 min | **Servings:** 4

INGREDIENTS:

salt and black pepper to taste

4 big tomatoes, halved and insides scooped out

1 tbsp. olive oil

½ tsp. thyme, chopped

2 garlic cloves, minced

DIRECTIONS:

In your air fryer, combine the tomatoes with the salt, pepper, oil, garlic and thyme, toss and bake at 390°F for fifteen minutes. Divide them between plates and serve as a garnish.

114. HOT TOMATOES MIX

Ready in about: 25 min | **Servings:** 8

INGREDIENTS:

4 garlic cloves, minced

1 jalapeno pepper, chopped

2 pounds cherry tomatoes, halved

¼ cup olive oil

¼ cup basil, chopped

salt and black pepper to taste

½ tsp. oregano, dried

DIRECTIONS:

In a portable bowl, combine the tomatoes with the garlic, jalapeño, salt, pepper, oregano, and oil, mix un
covered, transfer to the air fryer and cook at 380°F for 15 minutes. Divide the fried tomatoes between plate
sprinkle with basil and serve.

115. LEMONY ARTICHOKES

Ready in about: 25 min | **Servings:** 4

INGREDIENTS:

vegan cooking spray

2 medium artichokes, trimmed and halved

salt and black pepper to taste

2 tbsp. lemon juice

DIRECTIONS:

Grease your air fryer with cooking spray, add the artichokes, a little lemon juice, and a pinch of salt with bla
pepper and cook at 380°F for 15 minutes. Divide them among plates and serve as a garnish.

116. LEMONY BABY POTATOES

Ready in about: 35 min | **Servings:** 6

INGREDIENTS:

2 springs rosemary, chopped

2 tbsp. olive oil

2 tbsp. parsley, chopped

salt and black pepper to taste

1 tbsp. lemon rind, grated

2 tbsp. lemon juice

3 garlic cloves, minced

2 pounds baby potatoes

2 tbsp. oregano, chopped

DIRECTIONS:

In an enormous bowl, mix the new potatoes with the oil, rosemary, parsley, oregano, salt, pepper, lemon ze
garlic and lemon juice, mix, transfer apples of soil in the air fryer basket and bake at 356°F for 25 minut
Divide the potatoes between plates and serve.

117. MUSHROOM CAKES

Ready in about: 2 h 20 min | **Servings:** 8

INGREDIENTS:

- 1 small yellow onion, chopped
- 3½ ounces mushrooms, chopped
- salt and black pepper to taste
- 14 ounces of coconut milk
- 2 tbsp. olive oil
- ¼ tsp. nutmeg, ground
- 1 tbsp. vegan breadcrumbs

DIRECTIONS:

Heat a pan with half the oil over medium-high heat, add the onion and mushrooms, mix and cook for 3 minutes. Add the coconut milk. Add salt, pepper, and nutmeg, mix, remove from heat and let stand 2 hours. In a bowl, combine the remaining oil with the breadcrumbs and mix well. Take 1 tbsp. of mushroom filling, roll them in breadcrumbs and place them in the basket of your air fryer. Repeat with the rest of the mushroom mixture and bake the cakes at 400°F for 8 minutes. Divide the mushroom cakes between plates and serve.

118. POLENTA

Ready in about: 25 min | **Servings:** 4

INGREDIENTS:

- 3 cups water
- 1 cup cornmeal
- vegan cooking spray
- maple syrup for serving
- 1 tbsp. coconut oil

DIRECTIONS:

Pour the water for the polenta in a saucepan and heat over medium heat. Add the cornmeal, mix well and cook for 10 minutes. Add the oil, mix again, cook for another 2 minutes, remove from heat, let cool, take a tbsp. of polenta, form balls and place them in a lined pan. Use the cooking spray to grease the air fryer basket, add the polenta and cook for 16 minutes at 380°F, flipping them halfway. Serve with maple syrup on top.

119. ROASTED ASPARAGUS

Ready in about: 25 min | **Servings:** 4

INGREDIENTS:

- 1 tbsp. sweet paprika
- 1 pinch of salt and black pepper
- 1 lb. asparagus, trimmed
- 3 tbsp. olive oil

DIRECTIONS:

Take a bowl and mix the asparagus with the rest of the ingredients and mix. Place the asparagus in your air fryer basket and cook at 400°F for 10 minutes. Divide into plates and serve.

120. ROASTED EGGPLANT

Ready in about: 30 min | **Servings:** 6

INGREDIENTS:

- 1 tbsp. olive oil
- 1½ pounds eggplant, cubed
- 1 tsp. garlic powder
- 1 tsp. sumac
- 1 tsp. onion powder
- 2 tsp. za'atar
- 2 bay leaves
- juice from ½ lemon

DIRECTIONS:

In your air fryer, mix the eggplant cubes with olive oil, garlic powder, onion powder, sumac, za'atar, lemon juice, and bay leaves, stir and bake in the oven at 370°F for 20 minutes. Divide between plates and serve.

121. ROASTED PARSNIPS

Ready in about: 50 min | **Servings:** 6

INGREDIENTS:

- 2 pounds of peeled parsnips, cut into medium chunks
- 1 tbsp. parsley flakes, dried
- 2 tbsp. maple syrup
- 1 tbsp. olive oil

DIRECTIONS:

Warm your air fryer to 360°F, add oil, and heat it as well. Add the parsnips, parsley flakes, and maple syrup, mix and cook for 40 minutes. Divide between plates and serve.

122. ROASTED PEPPERS

Ready in about: 30 min | **Servings:** 4

INGREDIENTS:

- 1 tbsp. olive oil
- 1 tbsp. sweet paprika
- salt and black pepper to taste
- 4 green bell peppers, cut into medium strips
- 1 yellow onion, chopped

DIRECTIONS:

In your air fryer, mix the red peppers with green and yellow. Add paprika, oil, onion, salt, and pepper, mix and cook at 350°F for 20 minutes. Divide between the plates and serve.

123. ROASTED PUMPKIN

Ready in about: 22 min | **Servings:** 4

INGREDIENTS:

- 3 garlic cloves, minced
- 1½ pound pumpkin, deseeded, sliced and roughly chopped
- 1 pinch of cinnamon powder
- 1 tbsp. olive oil
- 1 pinch of brown sugar
- 1 pinch of sea salt
- 1 pinch of nutmeg, ground

DIRECTIONS:

In your air fryer basket, mix the pumpkin with the garlic, oil, salt, brown sugar, cinnamon and nutmeg, mix well, cover and cook at 370°F for 12 minutes. Divide between plates and serve.

124. SIMPLE POTATO CHIPS

Ready in about: 60 min | **Servings:** 4

INGREDIENTS:

- salt to taste
- 4 potatoes, scrubbed, peeled into thin chips,
- soaked in water for 30 minutes, drained and pat dried
- 2 tsp. rosemary, chopped
- 1 tbsp. olive oil

DIRECTIONS:

In a bowl, toss the fries with salt and oil to coat them, place them in the air fryer basket and bake at 330°F for minutes. Divide into plates, sprinkle with rosemary and serve.

125. SPICY CABBAGE

Ready in about: 18 min | **Servings:** 4

INGREDIENTS:

- 1 tbsp. sesame seed oil
- 1 cabbage, cut into 8 wedges
- 1 carrot, grated
- 1 tsp. red pepper flakes, crushed
- ¼ cups apple juice
- ¼ cup apple cider vinegar
- ½ tsp. cayenne pepper

DIRECTIONS:

In a pan suitable for your air fryer, combine the cabbage with the oil, carrot, vinegar, apple juice, cayenne pepper, and peppercorns, stir, place in the preheated air fryer and cook at 350°F for 8 minutes. Divide the cabbage mixture between plates and serve.

126. SWEET POTATO STUFFED

Ready in about: 1 h 10 min | **Servings:** 4

INGREDIENTS:

- 4 medium sweet potatoes
- 1 can chickpeas
- 1 tablespoon olive oil
- 1 cup ready to eat quinoa
- 1 teaspoon kosher salt

- 1/2 teaspoon black pepper
- 1/2 teaspoon cumin
- 1 cup baby spinach, roughly chopped
- 1 garlic clove, minced

- 2 tablespoons tahini
- parsley, chopped
- salt to taste
- crushed red pepper flakes

DIRECTIONS:

Preheat your Air Fryer to 375°F. Roast the potatoes for 50 minutes until just tender. Let them cool for 5 minut and halve them lengthwise. In the meantime, dry chickpeas and remove the skin. In a bowl toss the chickpe with oil, salt, pepper, and cumin. Cook them in a single layer for 25-30 minutes, until browned. While roasti chickpeas sauté the spinach for 3 minutes with garlic, salt, and pepper. Top the potato halves with spinach a quinoa under the chickpeas. Drizzle with tahini and sprinkle with salt and parsley.

127. YELLOW LENTILS MIX

Ready in about: 17 min | **Servings:** 4

INGREDIENTS:

- 1 cup yellow lentils, soaked in water for 1 hour and drained
- 1 hot chili pepper, chopped

- 1-inch ginger piece, grated
- 2 tsp. balsamic vinegar
- 2 tbsp. lime juice
- ½ tsp. turmeric powder

- 1 tsp. garam masala
- salt and black pepper to taste

DIRECTIONS:

In a pan suitable for your fryer, mix the olives with all the other ingredients, fry, put in the fryer and cook 12 minutes at 390°F. Divide the mixture between the plates and serve.

128. YELLOW SQUASH AND ZUCCHINIS

Ready in about: 45 min | **Servings:** 2

INGREDIENTS:

1 tbsp. tarragon, chopped
salt and white pepper to taste

1 yellow squash, halved, deseeded, and cut into chunks

1-pound zucchinis, sliced
6 tsp. olive oil
½ pound carrots, cubed

DIRECTIONS:

In your air fryer basket, toss zucchini with carrots, squash, salt, pepper, and oil, mix well and cook at 400°F for 25 minutes. Divide them among plates and serve as a garnish with a pinch of tarragon.

129. ZUCCHINI FRIES

Ready in about: 30 min | **Servings:** 4

INGREDIENTS:

1 tbsp. olive oil
3 zucchinis, cut into medium sticks

½ cup vegan breadcrumbs
¼ tsp. garlic powder

salt and black pepper to taste

DIRECTIONS:

In a portable bowl, combine the oil with the breadcrumbs, salt, pepper, and garlic powder and mix well. Coat the zucchini sticks with this mixture, place them in the basket of the air fryer, cover and bake at 425°F for 20 minutes. Divide them between plates and serve.

SNACK
AND
APPETIZERS

"One should not kill a living being, nor cause it to be killed, nor should one incite another to kill. Do not injure any being, either strong or weak, in the world."

— Buddha

130. AIR FRIED BANANA CHIPS

Ready in about: 30 min | **Servings:** 4

INGREDIENTS:

1 tsp. of vegetable oil
3 medium sized bananas, peeled

½ tsp. of Chaat masala seasoning
1 tsp. of salt

½ tsp. of Turmeric powder

DIRECTIONS:

Add about 1½ cups of water to the turmeric powder and a little salt. Cut the bananas in the turmeric mixtu
to prevent it from turning black and giving it a yellow color. Soak the bananas for 10 minutes, then drain ar
pat dry. Heat the air fryer to 356°F for 5 minutes. Add the oil to the fries and mix gently. Air Fry for 15 minut
in the air fryer. Remove from the fryer and add salt and seasoning. Serve immediately or store in an airtig
container.

131. BEANS SNACK

Ready in about: 15 min | **Servings:** 3

INGREDIENTS:

1 small can of beans
6 roll pastry (vegan)

2 tbsp. pineapple juice

2 tbsp. oil

DIRECTIONS:

Add the oil to the round pan. Mix the beans and pineapple juice with the puff pastry. Place the pan in the
fryer. Bake at 350°F for 10 minutes. When it's ready, help yourself and enjoy!

132. BEET CHIPS

Ready in about: 22 min | **Servings:** 5

INGREDIENTS:

14 ounces beets

½ tsp. olive oil

DIRECTIONS:

Peel the beets and cut them into chips. Then place the beet slices in the air fryer in a layer and sprinkle w
olive oil. Bake the beetroot fries for 14 minutes at 365°F. When the time is up and the fries are done, give
time to cool and serve.

133. CORN AND TOMATOES

Ready in about: 23 min | **Servings:** 4

INGREDIENTS:

4 tomatoes, roughly chopped

2 cups corn

1 tbsp. olive oil

1 tbsp. oregano, chopped

2 tbsp. soft tofu, pressed and crumbled

salt and black pepper to taste

1 tbsp. parsley, chopped

DIRECTIONS:

In a pan suitable for your air fryer, mix the corn with the tomatoes, oil, salt, pepper, oregano, and parsley, mix, place the pan in the air fryer and cook at 320°F for 10 minutes. Add the tofu, mix, place in the air fryer for another 3 minutes, divide between your plates and serve.

134. CORN TORTILLA CHIPS

Ready in about: 8 min | **Servings:** 3

INGREDIENTS:

8 corn tortillas

salt to taste

6 tsp. of vegetable oil

DIRECTIONS:

Heat the air fryer to 390°F. Cut out the shapes tortillas with a utility knife. Grease tortillas with oil using a pastry brush. Place half of the tortilla in the air fryer basket and cook for 3 minutes. Repeat a similar cycle with the subsequent batch until all the fries are done. Add salt and serve hot with the sauce.

135. CORN TORTILLAS MIX SNACK

Ready in about: 15 min | **Servings:** 3

INGREDIENTS:

3 cup coriander, chopped

1 tbsp. lime juice

2 tomatoes, diced

2 onion, sliced

2 tbsp. oil

10 corn tortillas

lime wedges to serve

DIRECTIONS:

Add oil into the air fryer pot. Combine cilantro, lime juice, tomato, corn tortillas, and onion. Cooking at 300°F 10 minutes. When finished, serve with lime wedges.

136. CREAMY ARTICHOKES

Ready in about: 16 min | **Servings:** 6

INGREDIENTS:

- 8 ounces coconut cream
- 14 ounces canned artichoke hearts
- 10 ounces spinach
- 3 garlic cloves, minced
- 1 tsp. onion powder
- ½ cup veggie stock
- ½ cup avocado mayonnaise

DIRECTIONS:

In a pan suitable for your air fryer, mix the artichokes with the broth, garlic, spinach, cream, onion powder and mayonnaise, stir, place in your air fryer and cook at 350°F for 6 minutes. Divide between plates and serve.

137. CREAMY GREEN BEANS AND WALNUTS

Ready in about: 25 min | **Servings:** 4

INGREDIENTS:

- 1 cup walnuts, chopped
- 1-pound green beans, trimmed and halved
- 2 cups cherry tomatoes, halved
- 1 tbsp. chives, chopped
- 1 pinch of salt and black pepper
- 2 tbsp. olive oil

DIRECTIONS:

Combine the green beans with nuts and other ingredients in a pan that fits the air fryer, mix, put the pan in the fryer and cook at 380°F for 20 minutes. Divide into plates and serve.

138. CREAMY ZUCCHINI AND SWEET POTATOES

Ready in about: 26 min | **Servings:** 8

INGREDIENTS:

- 2 tbsp. olive oil
- 1 cup veggie stock
- 2 peeled sweet potatoes, cut into medium wedges
- 2 yellow onions, chopped
- 8 zucchinis, cut into medium wedges
- 1 cup coconut milk
- 1 tbsp. coconut aminos
- salt and black pepper to taste
- ½ tsp. basil, chopped
- ¼ tsp. thyme, dried
- 4 tbsp. dill, chopped
- ¼ tsp. rosemary, dried

DIRECTIONS:

Heat a pan that fits in your air fryer with oil over medium heat, add the onion, mix and cook for 2 minutes. Add zucchini, thyme, rosemary, basil, potatoes, salt, pepper, broth, milk, amino acids a,nd dill, mix, place in air fryer, cook at 360°F for 14 minutes, divide into plates and serve.

139. CREAMY ZUCCHINIS

Ready in about: 24 min | **Servings:** 6

INGREDIENTS:

salt and black pepper to taste

6 zucchinis, halved and sliced

1 tbsp. olive oil

½ cup yellow onion, chopped

¾ cup coconut cream

1 tsp. oregano, dried

3 garlic cloves, minced

DIRECTIONS:

Heat a pan suitable for your air fryer with oil over medium-high heat, add the onion, stir and cook for 4 minutes. Add the garlic, zucchini, oregano, salt, pepper, and cream, mix, place in the air fryer and cook at 350°F for 10 minutes. Divide between plates and serve.

140. CRISPY FRENCH FRIES

Ready in about: 15 min | **Servings:** 2

INGREDIENTS:

2 tsp. olive oil

2 medium sweet potatoes

½ tsp. salt

black pepper to taste

¼ tsp. paprika

½ tsp. garlic powder

DIRECTIONS:

Set air-fryer temperature to 400°F. Sprig the air fryer basket with a little oil. Cut the sweet potatoes into shavings about 1 cm wide. Add the oil, salt, garlic powder, pepper, and paprika. Cook for 8 minutes, without overloading the basket. Repeat 2 or 3 times as needed.

141. CRUNCHY SWEET POTATO STICKS

Ready in about: 15 min | **Servings:** 1

INGREDIENTS:

salt to taste

1 tbsp. of vegan aioli

1 medium sized sweet potato

1 tsp. of coconut oil

DIRECTIONS:

Heat the air fryer to 280°F. Cut the sweet potatoes into sticks and add coconut oil. Place the potato sticks in the cooking basket and fry for 10 minutes until crispy. Add salt and serve with aioli.

142. DELICIOUS NUTS

Ready in about: 14 min | **Servings:** 3

INGREDIENTS:

- ¼ cup pistachios
- ¾ cup walnuts
- ½ tsp. salt
- 1 tsp. paprika
- ¼ tsp. olive oil

DIRECTIONS:

Place the nuts, pistachios, and salt in the air fryer basket; combine. Add the paprika and mix the mixture. The add the olive oil and shake the nut mixture well. Bake nuts at 320°F for 9 minutes, stirring halfway throug cooking. Let the cooked nuts cool to room temperature before serving.

143. EASY VEGAN FRITTATA

Ready in about: 20 min | **Servings:** 3

INGREDIENTS:

- 2 tbsp. flax meal mixed with 3 tbsp. water
- ½ vegan sausage, sliced
- 4 cherry tomatoes, halved
- salt and black pepper to taste
- 1 tbsp. olive oil
- 1 tbsp. parsley, chopped

DIRECTIONS:

Put the oil, tomatoes and vegan sausage in the pan of your air fryer, preheat to 360°F and cook for 5 minut Add the flax flour, parsley, salt, and pepper, mix, distribute in the pan, cover and cook at 360°F for anothe minutes. Cut, divide into plates and serve.

144. FLAVORED BEETS

Ready in about: 20 min | **Servings:** 4

INGREDIENTS:

- 1 drizzle of olive oil
- 1½ pounds beets, peeled and quartered
- 2 tsp. orange zest, grated
- ½ cup orange juice
- 2 tbsp. cider vinegar
- 2 tbsp. stevia
- 2 tsp. mustard
- 2 scallions, chopped

DIRECTIONS:

Rub the beets with the oil and orange juice, place them in the air fryer basket and bake at 350°F for 10 minut Transfer the beets to a bowl, add the shallot, orange zest, stevia, mustard, and vinegar, mix, divide into pla and serve.

145. GARLIC CARROTS

Ready in about: 25 min | **Servings:** 4

INGREDIENTS:

- 1-pound baby carrots, peeled
- 1 tbsp. avocado oil
- juice of 1 lime
- 6 garlic cloves, minced
- salt and black pepper to taste
- ½ tsp. sweet paprika
- 1 tbsp. balsamic vinegar

DIRECTIONS:

Combine carrots with oil and other ingredients in a pan that fits the air fryer, stir gently, place the pan in the air fryer and cook at 380°F for 20 minutes. Divide into plates and serve.

146. GARLIC CORN

Ready in about: 20 min | **Servings:** 4

INGREDIENTS:

- 3 garlic cloves, minced
- 2 cups corn
- 1 tbsp. olive oil
- 1 tsp. sweet paprika
- 2 tbsp. dill, chopped
- juice of 1 lime
- salt and black pepper to taste

DIRECTIONS:

Mix the corn with garlic and other ingredients in a suitable pan that fits your air fryer, stir, put the bread in the machine and bake at 390°F for 15 minutes. Divide everything between the plates and serve.

147. KALE AND BELL PEPPERS

Ready in about: 15 min | **Servings:** 4

INGREDIENTS:

- 2 cups kale, torn
- 1½ cups avocado, peeled, pitted, and cubed
- ¼ cup olive oil
- 1 tbsp. white vinegar
- 1 cup red bell pepper; sliced
- 2 tbsp. lime juice
- 1 pinch of salt and black pepper
- 1 tbsp. mustard

DIRECTIONS:

In a pan that fits the air fryer, mix the kale with the salt, pepper, avocado, and half the oil, mix. Spot in your air fryer and cook at 360°F for 10 minutes; in a bowl, mix the kale mixture with the rest of the ingredients, mix and serve.

148. KALE MIX SNACK

Ready in about: 15 min | **Servings:** 3

INGREDIENTS:

- 2 tbsp. oil
- 2 cups kale
- salt to taste
- 3 cup almonds, chopped
- 3 tbsp. lemon zest

DIRECTIONS:

Add oil into the air fryer pot. Combine the cabbage, salt, lemon zest, and almonds. Bake at 300°F for minutes. Serve.

149. LEMON TOMATOES

Ready in about: 25 min | **Servings:** 4

INGREDIENTS:

- 1 tsp. sweet paprika
- 2 pounds cherry tomatoes, halved
- 1 tsp. coriander, ground
- 2 tbsp. olive oil
- 1 handful parsley, chopped
- 2 tsp. lemon zest, grated
- 2 tbsp. lemon juice

DIRECTIONS:

Combine the tomatoes with the paprika and other ingredients in the air fryer pot, toss and bake at 370°F 20 minutes. Divide into plates and serve.

150. MILKY SCRAMBLED TOFU

Ready in about: 20 min | **Servings:** 4

INGREDIENTS:

- 2 tbsp. flax meal mixed with 2 tbsp. water
- 7 ounces almond milk
- 2 tbsp. firm tofu, crumbled
- 8 cherry tomatoes, cut into halves
- salt and black pepper to taste
- vegan cooking spray

DIRECTIONS:

In a bowl, combine the flax flour with the milk, salt, and pepper and mix well. Grease your air fryer with cook spray, pour in the flax flour, add the tofu, cook at 350°F for 6 minutes, stir a little and transfer to the plat Spread over the tomatoes and serve.

151. NUTS MIX SNACK

Ready in about: 15 min | **Servings:** 2

INGREDIENTS:

- 2 tbsp. oil
- 1 tbsp. garlic clove, minced
- 1 tbsp. paprika

- 3 tbsp. chili powder
- salt to taste
- 3 cup macadamia nuts

- 3 cup cashew nuts
- 1 tbsp. almond kernels
- 1 cup brazil nuts

DIRECTIONS:

Mix oil into the air fryer pot. Add the garlic clove, chili powder, paprika, salt, hazelnut almond, cashews, Brazil nuts, and macadamia nuts. Bake at 300°F for 10 minutes. Serve.

152. OLIVES AND SWEET POTATOES

Ready in about: 30 min | **Servings:** 4

INGREDIENTS:

- 1 cup Kalamata olives, pitted and halved
- 1-pound sweet potatoes, peeled and cut into wedges

- 1 tbsp. olive oil
- 1 bunch of cilantro, chopped
- 1 tbsp. basil, chopped

- 2 tbsp. balsamic vinegar
- salt and black pepper to taste

DIRECTIONS:

Combine the potatoes with olives and other ingredients and toss in a pan that fits the air fryer. Place the pan the air fryer. Cook at 370°F for 25 minutes. Divide into plates and serve!

153. OLIVES MIX APPETIZER

Ready in about: 20 min | **Servings:** 3

INGREDIENTS:

- 1 cup green olives
- 1 cup black olives
- 2 tbsp. lemon zest

- 2 garlic cloves, minced
- 2 tbsp. orange zest
- 1 onion, sliced

- thyme, chopped
- 1 tbsp. oil

DIRECTIONS:

Add oil into the air fryer pot. Combine black olives, green olives, lemon zest, orange zest, garlic cloves, onion, and thyme. Cook in your air fryer at 300°F for 15 minutes. Serve.

154. SESAME MUSTARD GREENS

Ready in about: 21 min | **Servings:** 6

INGREDIENTS:

- 1-pound mustard greens, torn
- 2 garlic cloves, minced
- 1 tbsp. olive oil
- salt and black pepper to taste
- ¼ tsp. dark sesame oil
- ½ cup yellow onion, sliced
- 3 tbsp. veggie stock

DIRECTIONS:

Heat a pan suitable for your air fryer with oil over medium heat, add the onions, stir and sauté for 5 minute Add garlic, broth, greens, salt, and pepper, mix, place in the air fryer and bake at 350°F for 6 minutes. Add t sesame oil, toss to coat, divide into plates and serve.

155. SIMPLE ONION

Ready in about: 20 min | **Servings:** 3

INGREDIENTS:

- 1¼ cups whole wheat flour
- 1 onion cut into medium slices and rings separated
- ¾ cup vegan breadcrumbs
- salt and black pepper to taste
- 1 tsp. baking powder
- 1 cup coconut milk

DIRECTIONS:

In a portable bowl, combine the flour with the salt and the baking powder and mix. Dip the onion rings in t flour and place them on a plate. Add milk to the flour mixture and mix well. Dip the onion rings in this mixtu roll them in breadcrumbs, put them in your air fryer, cook at 360°F for 10 minutes, divide them among t plates and serve as a garnish.

156. SIMPLE SMALL PEPPERS

Ready in about: 18 min | **Servings:** 8

INGREDIENTS:

- 1 tbsp. olive oil
- 3½ ounces cashew cheese, cubed
- 8 small bell peppers, tops cut off and seeds removed
- salt and black pepper to taste

DIRECTIONS:

In a bowl, combine the oil with salt and pepper and mix. Add the cashew cheese cubes and toss to coat. Pl a piece of cashew cheese on top of each pepper, put them all in your air fryer basket, and bake at 400°F fo minutes. Divide the peppers among plates and serve.

157. SIMPLE STUFFED TOMATOES

Ready in about: 25 min | **Servings:** 4

INGREDIENTS:

- salt and black pepper to taste
- 4 tomatoes, tops cut off and pulp scooped and chopped
- 1 yellow onion, chopped
- 2 tbsp. celery, chopped
- 1 tbsp. olive oil
- ½ cup mushrooms, chopped
- 1 cup cashew cheese
- 1 tbsp. parsley, chopped
- 1 tbsp. vegan breadcrumbs
- ¼ tsp. caraway seeds

DIRECTIONS:

Warmth up a saucepan with olive oil over medium heat, melt, add the onion and celery, mix and cook for 3 minutes. Add the chopped tomatoes and mushrooms, mix and cook for another 1 minute. Salt, pepper, crumbled bread, cashew cheese, cumin seeds, and parsley, mix, cook for another 4 minutes and remove from heat. Fill the tomatoes with this mixture, put them in your air fryer and cook at 350°F for 8 minutes. Divide the stuffed tomatoes among plates and serve.

158. TOMATOES AND BASIL MIX

Ready in about: 24 min | **Servings:** 2

INGREDIENTS:

- 3 garlic cloves, minced
- 1 bunch basil, chopped
- 1 drizzle of olive oil
- 2 cups cherry tomatoes, halved
- salt and black pepper to taste

DIRECTIONS:

In a pan suitable for your air fryer, combine the tomatoes with the garlic, salt, pepper, basil, and oil, mix, place in your air fryer and cook at 320°F for 12 minutes. Divide between plates and serve.

159. TOMATOES SALAD

Ready in about: 30 min | **Servings:** 2

INGREDIENTS:

- 1 green onion, chopped
- vegan cooking spray
- 2 tomatoes, halved
- salt and black pepper to taste
- 1 tsp. basil, chopped
- 1 tsp. parsley, chopped
- 1 tsp. oregano, chopped
- 1 cucumber, chopped
- 1 tsp. rosemary, chopped

DIRECTIONS:

Drizzle the tomato halves with the cooking oil, season with salt and pepper, place in the air fryer basket and bake at 320°F for 20 minutes. Transfer the tomatoes to a bowl, add the parsley, basil, oregano, rosemary, cucumber, and onion, toss and serve.

160. TORTILLA CHIPS

Ready in about: 15 min | **Servings:** 4

INGREDIENTS:

salt and black pepper to taste

8 corn tortillas, cut into triangles
1 tbsp. olive oil

1 pinch of sweet paprika
1 pinch of garlic powder

DIRECTIONS:

In a bowl, toss the tortilla chips with the oil, add salt, pepper, garlic powder and paprika, mix well, place in the air fryer basket and cook at 400°F for 6 minutes. Serve them as a garnish.

161. TURMERIC CABBAGE

Ready in about: 20 min | **Servings:** 4

INGREDIENTS:

¼ cup ghee; melted

1 green cabbage head, shredded

2 tsp. turmeric powder
1 tbsp. dill; chopped

DIRECTIONS:

In a pan that fits your air fryer, combine the cabbage with the rest of the ingredients except the dill, mix, place the pan in the air fryer and cook at 370°F for 15 minutes. Divide between plates and serve with dill sprinkled on top.

162. VEGAN VEGGIE DIP

Ready in about: 35 min | **Servings:** 4

INGREDIENTS:

1½ cups cauliflower florets
1 cup carrots, sliced
⅓ cup cashews
2½ cups water

½ cup turnips, chopped
1 cup almond milk
¼ cup nutritional yeast
1 tsp. garlic powder

¼ tsp. smoked paprika
¼ tsp. mustard powder
1 pinch of salt

DIRECTIONS:

In a pan that fits your air fryer, mix carrots with cauliflower, cashews, turnips, and water, stir, put in your fryer and cook at 365°F for 25 minutes. Transfer to a blender, add almond milk, garlic powder, yeast, paprika, mustard powder, and salt, blend well and serve.

163. ZUCCHINI AND OLIVES

Ready in about: 17 min | **Servings:** 4

INGREDIENTS:

2 tbsp. olive oil
4 zucchinis; sliced
1 cup Kalamata olives, pitted

salt and black pepper to taste
2 tsp. balsamic vinegar

2 tbsp. lime juice

DIRECTIONS:

In a pan suitable for your fryer, mix the olives with all the other ingredients, fry, put in the fryer and cook for 8 minutes at 390°F. Divide the mixture between the plates and serve.

164. ZUCCHINI BREAD

Ready in about: 45 min | **Servings:** 6

INGREDIENTS:

1½ banana, mashed
1 cup natural applesauce
1 tbsp. vanilla extract
2 cups zucchini, grated
4 tbsp. sugar

2½ cups coconut flour
vegan cooking spray
½ cup baking cocoa powder
¼ tsp. baking powder

½ cup walnuts, chopped
1 tsp. cinnamon powder
1 tsp. baking soda

DIRECTIONS:

Grease a loaf pan with cooking spray, add zucchini, sugar, vanilla, banana, applesauce, flour, cocoa powder, baking soda, baking powder, cinnamon, and walnuts, whisk well, introduce in the fryer and cook at 365°F for 30 minutes. Leave the bread to cool down, slice and serve.

165. ZUCCHINI CHIPS

Ready in about: 40 min | **Servings:** 6

INGREDIENTS:

3 zucchinis, thinly sliced
salt and black pepper to taste

2 tbsp. olive oil

2 tbsp. balsamic vinegar

DIRECTIONS:

In a portable bowl, mix oil with vinegar, salt, and pepper and whisk well. Add zucchini slices, toss to coat well, introduce in your air fryer and cook at 350°F for 30 minutes. Divide zucchini chips into bowls and serve them cold as a snack.

DESSERTS

*"Non-violence leads to the highest ethics,
which is the goal of all evolution. Until we stop harming
all other living beings, we are still savages."*

— Thomas A. Edison

166. AIR FRIED APPLES

Ready in about: 27 min | **Servings:** 4

INGREDIENTS:

1 handful raisin
agave nectar to the taste

4 big apples, cored

1 tbsp. cinnamon, ground

DIRECTIONS:

Fill each apple with raisins, sprinkle with cinnamon, a drizzle of agave nectar, put in the air fryer and cook 370°F for 17 minutes. Let cool and serve.

167. AIR FRIED PLANTAINS

Ready in about: 20 min | **Servings:** 4

INGREDIENTS:

2 ripened - almost brown – plantains

2 tsp. avocado or sunflower oil

⅛ tsp. salt

DIRECTIONS:

Heat the air fryer to 400°F. Slice the bananas at an angle 0.5 inches thick. Combine the oil, salt, and banana a bowl, making sure to cover the surface well. Set the timer for eight to ten minutes; shake after five minut If they don't suit you, add an extra minute or two. Serve.

168. ALMOND FLOUR

Ready in about: 20 min | **Servings:** 3

INGREDIENTS:

5 tbsp. almond flour
3 tbsp. cocoa powder
3 tbsp. sugar

1 tbsp. baking powder
3 tbsp. water
2 tbsp. avocado oil

¼ tsp. vanilla extract
1 pack vegan chocolate chips (sugar-free)

DIRECTIONS:

Add the flour and cocoa powder to the bowl. Mix sugar, yeast, water, avocado oil, and vanilla extract. Add chocolate chips. Pour the batter into the round pan. Bake at 300°F for 15 minutes in the air fryer. Serve a enjoy!

169. APPLE CAKE

Ready in about: 50 min | **Servings:** 6

INGREDIENTS:

- 1 cup coconut sugar
- 3 cups apples, cored and cubed
- 1 tbsp. vanilla extract

- 1 tbsp. apple pie spice
- 2 tbsp. flax meal combined with 3 tbsp. water
- 2 cups whole wheat flour

- 2 tbsp. vegetable oil
- 1 tbsp. baking powder

DIRECTIONS:

In a portable bowl, combine the flax flour with the oil, apple pie spice, apples, vanilla and sugar and mix with a mixer. In another portable bowl, mix the baking powder with the flour and mix. Combine the 2 mixtures, mix and pour into a spring form pan. Place the hinged pan in your air fryer and bake at 320°F for 40 minutes. Cut and serve.

170. APPLES AND MANDARIN SAUCE

Ready in about: 30 min | **Servings:** 4

INGREDIENTS:

- 2 cups mandarin juice
- 4 apples, cored, peeled, and cored

- ¼ cup maple syrup
- 1 tbsp. ginger, grated

- 2 tsp. cinnamon powder

DIRECTIONS:

In a pan suitable for your air fryer, mix the apples with the tangerine juice, maple syrup, cinnamon, and ginger, put them in the fryer and bake at 365°F for 20 minutes. Divide the apple mixture between plates and serve hot.

171. APPLES AND WINE SAUCE

Ready in about: 30 min | **Servings:** 2

INGREDIENTS:

- 1 tsp. nutmeg, ground
- ½ cup sugar

- 3 apples, cored and cut into wedges

- 1 cup red wine

DIRECTIONS:

In your air fryer's pan, combine the apples with the nutmeg and other ingredients, mix and cook at 340°F for minutes. Divide into bowls and serve.

172. BAKED PINEAPPLE DREAM

Ready in about: 20 min | **Servings:** 4

INGREDIENTS:

2 tbsp. agave nectar

2 tbsp. grated coconut

1 pineapple

1 tbsp. lime juice

DIRECTIONS:

First, cut the pineapple in half lengthwise. Remove the skin, deep seeds, and tough stalk from the pineapp Cut each half into 4 columns. Now mix the lime juice with the agave nectar in a bowl and brush the pineapp pieces. Place the pineapple boats in your air fryer and sprinkle with grated coconut. Bake everything for minutes at 180°F. A sorbet or a scoop of ice cream goes perfectly with this dessert.

173. BANANA S'MORES

Ready in about: 21 min | **Servings:** 3

INGREDIENTS:

3 tbsp. mini-peanut butter chips

3 tbsp. vegan chocolate chips - semi-sweet

4 bananas

3 tbsp. Graham cracker cereal

DIRECTIONS:

Heat the air fryer to 400°F in advance. Slice the unpeeled bananas along the inside of the curve. Do not cut t base of the shell. Open slightly, forming a pocket. Fill each pocket with peanut butter flakes and chocol. chips. Put the grains in the filling. Place the stuffed plantains in the air fryer basket, holding them upright w the stuffing facing up. Air fry until skin is black and chocolate is toasted (6 minutes). Let it cool for 1 tc minutes. Spread out the filling to serve.

174. BERRIES MIX

Ready in about: 11 min | **Servings:** 4

INGREDIENTS:

1½ tbsp. maple syrup

2 tbsp. lemon juice

1½ tbsp. champagne vinegar

¼ cup basil leaves, torn

1-pound strawberries, halved

1 tbsp. olive oil

1½ cups blueberries

DIRECTIONS:

In a pan suitable for your air fryer, combine the lemon juice with the maple syrup and vinegar, bring to a b over medium-high heat, add the oil, blueberries, strawberries, mix, add to the air fryer and bake at 310°F fo minutes. Sprinkle with basil and serve!

175. BLUEBERRY BOWLS

Ready in about: 22 min | **Servings:** 4

INGREDIENTS:

1 cup coconut water

2 cups blueberries

2 tbsp. sugar

juice of ½ lime

2 tsp. vanilla extract

DIRECTIONS:

your air fryer's pan, mix the blueberries with the water and the other ingredients, mix and cook at 320°F for minutes. Serve cold.

176. CHOCOLATE BANANA

Ready in about: 12 min | **Servings:** 2

INGREDIENTS:

10 vegan chocolate chips

2 bananas

DIRECTIONS:

Use a knife to cut the banana deeply lengthwise. Be careful, however, not to completely cut the banana. Now the chocolate chips in this slot. Place the plantains in the coated pan of your air fryer and bake for 6 minutes 350°F. Cut the banana into small pieces and serve.

177. CINNAMON APPLES

Ready in about: 20 min | **Servings:** 4

INGREDIENTS:

5 apples, cored and cut into chunks

2 tsp. cinnamon powder

½ tsp. nutmeg powder

½ cup water

1 tbsp. maple syrup

4 tbsp. vegetable oil

¼ cup coconut sugar

¾ cup old-fashioned rolled oats

¼ cup whole wheat flour

DIRECTIONS:

Place the apples in a saucepan suitable for your air fryer, add the cinnamon, nutmeg, maple syrup and water. Add the oil mixed with oats, sugar, and flour, mix, spread over the apples, place in the air fryer, cook at 350°F 10 minutes and serve hot.

178. CINNAMON ROLLS

Ready in about: 2 h 15 min | **Servings:** 8

INGREDIENTS:

- ¾ cup coconut sugar
- 2 tbsp. vegetable oil
- 1-pound vegan bread dough
- 1½ tbsp. cinnamon powder

DIRECTIONS:

Spin out the dough on a floured work surface, form a rectangle and brush with oil. In a bowl, mix the cinnamon with the sugar, stir, sprinkle the dough on the dough, roll into a log, seal well and cut into 8 pieces. Let the rolls rise for 2 hours, place in the air fryer basket, bake at 350°F for 5 minutes, flip, bake another 4 minutes and transfer to a serving plate.

179. COCOA AND ALMOND BARS

Ready in about: 34 min | **Servings:** 6

INGREDIENTS:

- 1 cup almonds, soaked and drained
- ¼ cup cocoa nibs
- 2 tbsp. cocoa powder
- 8 dates, pitted and soaked
- ¼ cup goji berries
- ¼ cup hemp seeds
- ¼ cup coconut, shredded

DIRECTIONS:

Put the almonds in your food processor, mix, add hemp seeds, the cocoa nibs, cocoa powder, goji, coconut, and mix well. Add the dates, mix well again, spread on a lined baking sheet that fits your air fryer, and bake 320°F for 4 minutes. Cut into equal parts and refrigerate 30 minutes before serving.

180. COFFEE PUDDING

Ready in about: 20 min | **Servings:** 4

INGREDIENTS:

- 4 ounces dark vegan chocolate, chopped
- 4 ounces coconut butter
- juice of ½ orange
- 2 ounces whole wheat flour
- 1 tsp. baking powder
- ½ tsp. instant coffee
- 2 ounces coconut sugar
- 2 tbsp. flax meal combined with 2 tbsp. water

DIRECTIONS:

Heat a pan with coconut butter over medium heat, add the chocolate and orange juice, mix well and remove from the heat. In a bowl, mix the sugar with the instant coffee and the flax flour, beat with a mixer, add the chocolate mixture, the flour, the salt and the baking powder and mix well. Pour into a greased pan, place in your air fryer, cook at 360°F for 10 minutes, divide into plates and serve.

181. EASY DONUTS

eady in about: 25 min | **Servings:** 4

INGREDIENTS:

- 2 tbsp. coconut sugar
- 8 ounces whole wheat flour
- 1 tbsp. flax meal mixed with 2 tbsp. water
- 1 tsp. baking powder
- 4 ounces almond milk
- 2½ tbsp. vegetable oil

DIRECTIONS:

In a portable bowl, mix 1 tbsp. of oil with the sugar, baking powder, and flour and mix. In a second bowl, combine the flax flour with 1½ tbsp. of oil and milk and mix well. Combine the 2 mixtures, mix, form donuts from this mixture, put them in the basket of the air fryer and cook at 360°F for 15 minutes. Serve hot.

182. EASY GRANOLA

eady in about: 45 min | **Servings:** 4

INGREDIENTS:

- ½ cup almonds
- 1 cup coconut, shredded
- ½ cup pecans, chopped
- ½ cup pumpkin seeds
- 2 tbsp. sugar
- ½ cup sunflower seeds
- 1 tsp. apple pie spice mix
- 1 tsp. nutmeg, ground
- 2 tbsp. sunflower oil

DIRECTIONS:

In an enormous bowl, combine the almonds and nuts with pumpkin seeds, the sunflower seeds, coconut, nutmeg and mix pie spice apple and mix well. Heat a pan with the oil over medium heat, add the sugar and mix well. Pour it over the nuts and coconut and mix well. Unfurl it out on a lined baking sheet that fits your air fryer, put it in your fryer, and bake at 300°F and bake for 25 minutes. Let the granola cool, cut and serve.

183. EASY PEARS DESSERT

eady in about: 35 min | **Servings:** 12

INGREDIENTS:

- ½ cup raisins
- 6 big pears, cored and chopped
- 1 tsp. ginger powder
- 1 tsp. lemon zest, grated
- ¼ cup coconut sugar

DIRECTIONS:

In a saucepan suitable for your air fryer, mix the pears with the raisins, ginger, sugar, and lemon zest, mix, place in the air fryer and bake at 350°F for 25 minutes. Divide into bowls and serve cold.

184. FIGS AND COCONUT BUTTER MIX

Ready in about: 10 min | **Servings:** 3

INGREDIENTS:

12 figs, halved

1 cup almonds, toasted and chopped

2 tbsp. coconut butter

¼ cup sugar

DIRECTIONS:

Place the butter in a pan suitable for your air fryer and melt over medium-high heat. Add figs, sugar, an almonds, mix, place in the fryer and cook at 300°F for 4 minutes. Divide into bowls and serve cold.

185. GRAPE PUDDING

Ready in about: 50 min | **Servings:** 6

INGREDIENTS:

3 cups grapes

1 cup grapes curd

3½ ounces maple syrup

2 ounces coconut butter, melted

3 tbsp. flax meal combined with 3 tbsp. water

3½ ounces almond milk

½ tsp. baking powder

½ cup almond flour

DIRECTIONS:

In a bowl, mix half the fruit curd with the grapes, mix and divide into 6 heat-resistant mussels. In a bowl, m the flax flour with the maple syrup, the melted coconut butter, the rest of the curd, the baking powder, t milk, and the flour and mix well. Divide it into the molds, place it in the air fryer and bake at 400°F for minutes. Let the puddings cool and serve!

186. LEMON SQUARES

Ready in about: 40 min | **Servings:** 6

INGREDIENTS:

½ cup vegetable oil

1 cup whole wheat flour

1¼ cups coconut sugar

2 tsp. lemon peel, grated

1 medium banana

2 tbsp. lemon juice

½ tsp. baking powder

2 tbsp. flax meal combine with 2 tbsp. water

DIRECTIONS:

In a portable bowl, combine the flour with ¼ cup of sugar and oil, mix well, press on the bottom of a saucep suitable for your air fryer, place in the air fryer and bake at 350°F for 14 minutes. In another portable bo mix the rest of the sugar with the lemon juice, lemon zest, banana, and yeast, mix with the blender. Spre over the baked crust. Bake for another 15 minutes, let cool, cut into medium squares and serve cold.

187. LENTILS AND DATES BROWNIES

Ready in about: 25 min | **Servings:** 8

INGREDIENTS:

12 dates

28 ounces canned lentils, rinsed and drained

1 tbsp. agave nectar

½ tsp. baking soda

2 tbsp. cocoa powder

1 banana, peeled and chopped

4 tbsp. almond butter

DIRECTIONS:

In your food processor, mix the lentils with the butter, banana, cocoa, baking soda, and agave nectar and mix very well. Add the dates, mix a few times again, pour into a greased pan suitable for your air fryer, distribute evenly, place in the air fryer at 360°F and bake for 15 minutes. Take the brownies out of the oven, slice them, place them in a serving dish and serve.

188. ORANGE BREAD

Ready in about: 60 min | **Servings:** 8

INGREDIENTS:

juice of 2 oranges

1 orange, peeled and sliced

3 tbsp. vegetable oil

¾ cup almonds, ground

¾ cup coconut sugar+ 2 tbsp.

2 tbsp. flax meal combined with 2 tbsp. water

¾ cup whole wheat flour

DIRECTIONS:

Grease a loaf pan with a drizzle of oil, sprinkle 2 tbsp. of sugar and place the orange slices at the bottom. In a bowl, mix the oil with ¾ cup of sugar, almonds, flour, and orange juice, mix, pour the orange slices on top, place the pan in the air fryer and cook at 360°F for 40 minutes. Cut and serve the bread immediately.

189. ORANGE CAKE

Ready in about: 40 min | **Servings:** 4

INGREDIENTS:

1 tsp. baking powder

vegan cooking spray

1 cup almond flour

½ tsp. cinnamon powder

1 cup coconut sugar

3 tbsp. coconut oil, melted

½ cup pecans, chopped

½ cup almond milk

¾ cup water

¾ cup orange juice

½ cup orange peel, grated

½ cup raisins

DIRECTIONS:

In an enormous bowl, mix the flour with half the sugar, baking powder, cinnamon, 2 tbsp. of oil, milk, nuts and raisins, mix and pour into a greased pan suitable for your air fryer. Heat a saucepan over medium heat, add the water, orange juice, orange zest, the rest of the oil, and the rest of the sugar, mix, bring to a boil, pour the mixture from the pan over an air fryer and cook at 330°F for 30 minutes. Serve cold.

190. PEACH COBBLER

Ready in about: 40 min | **Servings:** 4

INGREDIENTS:

¼ cup coconut sugar

4 cups peaches, peeled and sliced

½ tsp. cinnamon powder

¼ cup stevia

1½ cups vegan crackers, crushed

vegan cooking spray

¼ tsp. nutmeg, ground

1 tsp. vanilla extract

½ cup almond milk

DIRECTIONS:

In a portable bowl, combine the peaches with the coconut sugar and cinnamon and mix. In another bowl, to the cookies with stevia, nutmeg, almond milk, and vanilla extract and mix. Spray a cake pan suitable for yo air fryer with cooking spray and sprinkle the peaches on the bottom. Add the cookies, toss, spread, place in t air fryer and bake at 350°F for 30 minutes. Divide the cobbler among the plates and serve.

191. PEAR STEW

Ready in about: 30 min | **Servings:** 4

INGREDIENTS:

4 pears, cored and cut into wedges

2 tbsp. sugar

2 tsp. cinnamon powder

1 cup water

DIRECTIONS:

In your air fryer's pan, combine the pears with the water and other ingredients, cook at 300°F for 20 minut divide into cups and serve cold.

192. QUINOA PUDDING

Ready in about: 30 min | **Servings:** 6

INGREDIENTS:

1 tsp. vanilla extract

2 cups almond milk

1 tsp. nutmeg, ground

½ cup sugar

1 cup quinoa

DIRECTIONS:

In your air fryer pan, mix the almond milk with the quinoa and other ingredients, whisk and cook at 320°F 20 minutes. Divide into bowls and serve.

193. SIMPLE AND SWEET BANANAS

Ready in about: 25 min | **Servings:** 4

INGREDIENTS:

- 2 tbsp. flax meal combined with 2 tbsp. water
- 3 tbsp. coconut butter
- 4 bananas, peeled and halved
- 1 cup vegan breadcrumbs
- 3 tbsp. cinnamon powder
- ½ cup corn flour

DIRECTIONS:

Heat a pan with butter over medium-high heat, add the breadcrumbs, mix and cook for 4 minutes, then transfer to a bowl. Roll each banana in flour, flax flour, and breadcrumbs. Spot the bananas in the air fryer basket, sprinkle with cinnamon sugar, and cook at 280°F for 10 minutes. Transfer to plates and serve.

194. SIMPLE GELATIN

Ready in about: 20 min | **Servings:** 4

INGREDIENTS:

- 3 packs gelatin
- 2 tbsp. sugar
- 2 tbsp. corn syrup
- 2 tbsp. vanilla extract
- powdered sugar for dusting
- 2 cups strawberries, sliced

DIRECTIONS:

Add the gelatin and sugar to the bowl. Combine the corn syrup, vanilla extract, and strawberries. Pour the batter into the round pan. Bake at 300°F for 15 minutes in the air fryer. When you are ready, sprinkle with sugar to serve!

195. STRAWBERRY COBBLER

Ready in about: 35 min | **Servings:** 6

INGREDIENTS:

- 6 cups strawberries, halved
- ¾ cup sugar
- ⅛ tsp. baking powder
- ½ cup flour
- 1 tbsp. lemon juice
- vegan cooking spray
- 1 pinch of baking soda
- 3½ tbsp. olive oil
- ½ cup water

DIRECTIONS:

In an enormous bowl, mix the strawberries with half the sugar, sprinkle with a little flour, add the lemon juice, heat and pour into the appropriate pot for your air fryer and greased with cooking spray. In another bowl, combine the flour with the remaining sugar, baking powder, and soda and mix well. Include olive oil and mix until everything is done with your hands. Add ½ cup of water and sprinkle over the strawberries. Place in the fryer at 355°F and bake for 25 minutes. Let the cobbler cool, slice and serve.

196. SWEET BANANAS AND SAUCE

Ready in about: 30 min | **Servings:** 4

INGREDIENTS:

3 tbsp. agave nectar
juice of ½ lemon
1 tbsp. coconut oil

½ tsp. cardamom seeds

4 bananas, peeled and
sliced diagonally

DIRECTIONS:

Place the plantains in your air fryer, add the agave nectar, lemon juice, oil, and cardamom, place in the air fry
and cook at 360°F for 20 minutes. Divide the plantains and the sauce between the plates and serve.

197. SWEET CASHEW STICKS

Ready in about: 25 min | **Servings:** 6

INGREDIENTS:

¼ cup almond meal
⅓ cup stevia
1 tbsp. almond butter

4 dates, chopped
1 tbsp. chia seeds
1½ cups cashews, chopped

¾ cup coconut, shredded

DIRECTIONS:

In a bowl, combine the stevia with the almond flour, almond butter, cashews, coconut, dates, and chia see
and mix well again. Spread it out on a lined baking sheet that fits your fryer, press down well, put it in the ;
fryer, and bake at 300°F for 15 minutes. Let the dough cool, cut it into medium sticks and serve.

198. SWEET STRAWBERRY MIX

Ready in about: 30 min | **Servings:** 10

INGREDIENTS:

- 2 pounds strawberries
- 2 tbsp. lemon juice

- 4 cups coconut sugar
- 1 tsp. vanilla extract

- 1 tsp. cinnamon powd

DIRECTIONS:

In a portable pan that fits your air fryer, mix the strawberries with the coconut sugar, lemon juice, cinnam
and vanilla, mix gently, place in the air fryer and cook at 350°F for 20 minutes. Divide into bowls and ser
cold.

199. SWEET TOMATO BREAD

Ready in about: 40 min | **Servings:** 4

INGREDIENTS:

1 tsp. cinnamon powder

1½ cups whole wheat flour

1 tsp. baking powder

¾ cup maple syrup

1 tsp. baking soda

1 cup tomatoes, chopped

2 tbsp. apple cider vinegar

½ cup olive oil

DIRECTIONS:

In a portable bowl, combine the flour with the baking powder, baking soda, cinnamon, and maple syrup and mix well. In another bowl, combine the tomatoes with olive oil and vinegar and mix well. Combine the 2 mixtures, mix well, pour into a greased pan that suits your air fryer, put in the air fryer and cook at 360°F for 30 minutes. Let the cake cool, slice it and serve.

200. TOMATO CAKE

Ready in about: 50 min | **Servings:** 6

INGREDIENTS:

1 pound tomatoes

½ cup brown sugar, packed

½ cup granulated sugar

¾ cup coconut butter, softened

4 tbsp. cornstarch

2 cups all-purpose flour

2 teaspoons baking powder

1 teaspoon baking soda

1 teaspoon salt

1 teaspoon ground cinnamon

1 teaspoon ground cardamom

½ teaspoon ground ginger

1½ cup powdered sugar

½ teaspoon pure vanilla extract

DIRECTIONS:

Preheat the oven to 350°F and grease a pan with vegan cooking spray. Core tomatoes and quarter. Purée in a blender until completely smooth. Measure out two cups and set aside, reserving remainder. In a large bowl, beat together brown sugar, granulated sugar, and coconut butter until creamed and fluffy. Add cornstarch and mix. In another bowl, mix together flour, baking powder, baking soda, salt, cinnamon, cardamom, and ginger. Alternate adding flour mixture and tomato purée to the batter, starting and ending with the flour. Pour batter into prepared pan and bake for 40 minutes, or until a toothpick comes out clean. Let cake cool in pan 10 minutes, then invert onto a rack and cool completely. To make the glaze, mix together powdered sugar, vanilla, and 2-3 tablespoons leftover tomato juice until completely smooth. Add more sugar or liquid as necessary. Drizzle over cooled cake and serve.

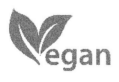

...sso ...aso ...mm	Kern fond int. núcleo ∅ mm	trap mèche broca ∅ mm
		2.5
	2.46	3.
0.5	3.24	4.
0.7	4.13	
0.8	4.92	
1	6.65	

APPENDIX WITH CONVERSION MEASURE

WEIGHTS	
IMPERIAL	**METRIC**
½ oz.	15 g
¾ oz.	20 g
1 oz.	30 g
2 oz.	60 g
3 oz.	85 g

16 oz. = 1 pound= 435 g

1 oz. = 28.35 g | 1 g = 0.035 oz.

COMMON INGREDIENTS

1 CUP	IMPERIAL	METRIC
Flour	5 oz.	140 g
Almonds	4 oz.	110 g
Uncooked Rice	6½ oz.	190 g
Brown Sugar	6½ oz.	185 g
Raisins	7 oz.	200 g

LIQUIDS

CUPS	METRIC	PINT	QUART
¼	60 ml	-	-
½	125 ml	-	-
-	150 ml	¼	-
-	200 ml	-	-
1	250 ml	½	-
-	300 ml	-	-
-	400 ml	-	-
2	500 ml	-	-
-	950 ml	-	1

OVEN TEMPS

°F	°C
250	120
275	140
300	150
325	170
350	180
375	190
400	200

SPOONS

LIQUID		DRY	
¼ tsp.	1.25 ml	¼ tsp.	1.1 g
½ tsp.	2.5 ml	½ tsp.	2.3 g
1 tsp.	5 ml	1 tsp.	4.7 g
¼ tbsp.	3.75 ml	¼ tbsp.	3.5 g
½ tbsp.	7.5 ml	½ tbsp.	7.1 g
1 tbsp.	15 ml	1 tbsp.	14.3 g

INGREDIENT INDEX

RECIPE INDEX

Side Dishes 53

Printed in Great Britain
by Amazon